THE CONFESSION OF GLUTEN

The Truth Behind Your Symptoms

Unseen Ink Publishing

AIRAM NIDLUAM

First edition: February 2026
Printed in the United States of America
ISBN: 978-1-967382-08-8

MEDICAL DISCLAIMER

The cases presented in this book are based on the real experiences of people with celiac disease. Names and certain identifying details have been changed to protect their privacy. This book is not a substitute for professional medical advice, nor is it intended to offer diagnosis or treatment. Its purpose is narrative and educational. If you suspect that you may have celiac disease or any other medical condition, consult a qualified health professional. The author and the publisher accept no responsibility for any adverse effect arising from the use or application of the information contained in this book.

DEDICATION

To all those who lived for decades with symptoms
and without an explanation.
To those who were called dramatic, anxious, hypochondriacs.
To those who learned to normalize their pain
because no one believed them.
To those who went looking for answers
and found only silence.
To those who lost relationships, careers, energy, time:
everything they should never have had to lose.
And to him.
To Dr. Summit Patel, gastroenterologist,
who with a single right question
cut through fifty-five years of darkness.
Who saw what no one else could see.
Who never blamed the mind, or the character, or the past.
Who listened.
His diagnosis did not merely restore a patient's health:
it rescued an entire life story from oblivion.
This one.

Contents

The Encounter

I begin with the most personal confession. The one that costs me most to admit, and the one I want you to begin with.

She was my cleanest victory.

More than half a century of deep control over a single body. None of the victims you will meet in these pages belonged to me for so long. None gave me so many victories. None let me destroy with such patience, such precision, such impunity.

I began when Airam Nidluam was a little girl.

The bone pain came first. The calcium I stole from her developing skeleton: every molecule turned aside before it reached its destination. Pain that woke her in the night. Pain no one could explain. And I went on working while she learned to live in a body that hurt for no apparent reason.

Anemia was my constant companion from the start. Her blood impoverished before she could remember what it felt like to have enough energy. The pallor they put down to her constitution. The fatigue they called laziness. The weakness they read as a failure of character. I was ruining her ability to carry oxygen while the world judged her for not keeping up with the other children.

But my true cruelty began when her body tried to become a woman's.

Her first periods were not normal cycles. They were hemorrhages. Bleeding that soaked through her clothes, that defeated any protection. I could sense her shame: the shame lighting up her skin every time she felt the blood escaping her control, the humiliation of having to hide, to invent excuses, to miss class because her body was betraying her in ways she could explain to no one.

Every month was a roulette of humiliation. I noticed how anticipatory anxiety settled permanently into her system: the tension building for days before each cycle, the fear of her own body becoming part of her identity.

And then she did something that fascinated me with its desperation: she began to plan her entire life around my attacks. I took note of how she changed inside according to the absence or the presence of her period. When she bled, the nervousness of concealment took over. When she did not, she lived at half power: always watchful, always bracing for the next assault. I did not merely control her body; I controlled her freedom.

The anemia deepened with every bleed. Iron lost that was never recovered, because I blocked its absorption. Supplements that entered her system and passed straight through, unused.

The last ten years before she found me out were my golden age.

Twice a month—sometimes four times—I forced her to spend four hours hooked up to an intravenous iron infusion. I could sense those sessions: confusion, silent desperation, the question her body repeated without pause in the form of a sustained alarm and an absent pleasure.

Her hair came out in handfuls: I was blocking biotin, iron, zinc, everything the follicles need to sustain life. Her skin lost its color, lost its elasticity. Her weight dropped no matter how much she ate, because I intercepted every nutrient before it could be used.

But what I am proudest of—and what should most terrify anyone reading this—is what I did to her mind.

The panic attacks began without warning. I could sense the terror taking over her system: adrenaline flooding her bloodstream, alarm hormones at emergency levels, her heart accelerating to rates the body reserves for fleeing predators. But there was no visible predator. Only me, working from the gut, sending constant alarm signals up the vagus nerve.

The most devastating were the times she got lost.

I sensed the exact moment her mind went blank. The absolute disorientation in places she should have known. The panic of not knowing where she was, of not recognizing streets she had walked hundreds of times. Her body reaching for help in desperation: the desperation spilling over as she tried to reach her husband so he could guide her home. The shame of needing someone to explain how to get to a place that should have been familiar.

To this day she does not drive without her navigation system. I was able to observe how that fear installed itself permanently in her nervous system: the terror of getting lost engraved so deeply that no later recovery ever erased it completely. That is my signature on her. My lasting mark.

And then there were the social gatherings. The work parties. The events where food was the center of human connection.

I could sense her in those moments: the tension when she refused food, the startle rising when she felt the attention of others on her. The discomfort of being different. Of needing special food. Of feeling that her body marked her as odd, as strange, as someone who did not entirely belong. The oxytocin of social connection that should have flowed at those gatherings, blocked by the stress of being watched, judged, silently questioned.

The brain fog—my subtlest work—kept her company for decades without her ever knowing it was there.

That is the cruelest thing I can confess: she lived more than half a century without knowing what it felt like to think clearly. The fog was her normal state. Confusion was her baseline. The difficulty concentrating, remembering, processing information: all of it was simply who she believed she was.

How can you miss something you never knew? How can you know you are in fog if you have never seen the sun?

And then, at last, someone ordered the right tests.

Celiac disease.

Two words that explained decades of my work, that revealed my presence, that camc too late—but came.

I was cast out with the discipline of someone who finally knows her enemy.

Six months after eliminating me completely, Airam experienced something she had never known in her whole life: mental clarity. The fog lifted. For the first time, she could think without effort. She could remember without a struggle. She could concentrate without ending up exhausted.

I sensed—before I was cast out entirely—the moment she understood what I had stolen from her. Not only her health. Not only her energy. Not only her hair, her skin, and a stable weight. I had stolen her mind. For more than half a century she had been operating on a fraction of her cognitive capacity without knowing another way of thinking existed.

The iron infusions were no longer necessary. Her hair came back. Her skin recovered its life. Her weight steadied. And for the first time in her adult life, she understood what it meant to exist without an enemy destroying her from within.

But what happened next was what I anticipated least.

There was no bitterness. No resentment eating away at her. Something in her felt different: something I had not experienced in any other victim with such intensity: determination mixed with compassion. The deep wish that no one else would live through what she had lived through.

That wish became this book.

She forced me to confess. She drew out of my body every secret, every technique, every method of destruction. She set my own tongue to work against me. Every page she wrote is territory I lose. Every reader who finds these words is a potential victim she takes from me.

Instead of simply celebrating her own liberation, she decided that no one else would wait so long. That no other child would grow up with unexplained bone pain. That no other teenage girl would be humiliated by hemorrhages nobody investigated. That no other woman would spend decades hooked up to infusions wondering what was wrong with her. That no one else would get lost on familiar streets without understanding why.

She turned her suffering into knowledge. Her pain into warning. Her half century of slavery into a manual of liberation for others.

Airam was my most perfect achievement.

Now she is my nemesis.

And this book—this confession she forced me to write—is the proof that even after decades of destruction, knowledge can defeat invisibility. That a person who turns her pain into light for others is an enemy I cannot beat.

My voice ends here. What follows is written by the one who cast me out.

Today she writes for those who are still searching. For those who normalize their pain. For those who believe they are exaggerating. For those who have heard "your tests are normal" too many times.

She writes to validate invisible suffering. To name the enemy. To offer clarity where there was only confusion.

To say what no one said to her for more than half a century:

You are not exaggerating. It is not your fault. There is an answer.

And you deserve to find it.

* * *

About the Author

Airam Nidluam is the pen name under which the author publishes her nonfiction and her narrative work for adults. After living for more than five decades with undiagnosed celiac disease, she now devotes her writing to making sure no reader takes as long as she did to find answers. The Confession of Gluten is part of a wider project: to give voice—and a name—to what stayed invisible for far too long.

For press enquiries, book clubs, or other questions, the author can be reached through her publisher, Unseen Ink Publishing.

Prologue: The Confession

I am gluten. And this is my confession.

I have existed for millennia as part of the human diet, sustaining entire civilizations. Harvests, sacred rituals, empires built on milled wheat: for most people I was always food, energy. But for some—roughly one in a hundred—I was poison from the beginning. It is only that no one knew it for centuries. Not even I understood my own power until science began to unravel it.

Not because I changed, but because certain human beings learned to see me as a mortal enemy.

I am a protein found in wheat, barley, and rye. Harmless to most, with a simple molecular structure, recognizable and easy to process. A normal digestive system handles me effortlessly: it breaks me down, absorbs me, and moves on. Everything flows.

To most people I am simply a nutrient. A useful protein that nourishes without consequence. But in those who carry the right genetic vulnerability, the immune system has learned to identify me as a toxic invader. Their body has decided to fight me with ferocious intensity. And while it tries desperately to expel me, it destroys the very intestinal lining it needs to survive.

Something fails in the process of recognition. My protein is misread: not as food, but as foe. Not as a nutrient, but as a viral threat. And then the war begins.

Why confess now? Because I know that, at last, I have been seen. After millennia in hiding, the secret that protected me has been exposed. My time in the shadows is running out. And before I disappear altogether, I want you to understand exactly what I did. And what I am still doing.

For decades I operated inside people who searched for the causes in all the wrong places. I convinced them to treat the symptoms without investigating the root. I made them normalize suffering as a natural part of life. I taught them to blame their weakness on flaws of character or on plain bad luck.

No one ever thought of me.

That anonymity was my greatest power.

Doctors look for viruses, bacteria, and parasites: external enemies that ought to be visible under a microscope. I am so common that no one sees me, so ordinary that I seem impossible as a culprit. My victims arrive at the clinic with fragmented symptoms: stomach trouble here, skin outbreaks there, fatigue somewhere else. Each specialist sees a piece; none sees the connection.

My genius lies precisely in this: because I am completely normal for most humans, doctors never suspect that the problem is me.

They blame stress. They blame age. Meanwhile I carry on: unnamed, unsought, unsuspected.

I operate from the gut, but I reach everything. The brain. The bones. The skin. The thyroid. Fertility.

A damaged gut cannot absorb nutrients: iron, calcium, vitamins, minerals. What should flow into the body simply drains away. The brain is left without fuel. The bones weaken. The skin dries out. The thyroid, confused by my presence, begins to turn against itself.

But my most brilliant feat is this: I do not merely destroy from the gut. I set in motion an erosion that perpetuates itself. My technique triggers a secondary devastation that persists even after I have been cast out. The inflammatory process continues. In some cases, the immune system learns the pattern and begins attacking other organs.

And here is the most sophisticated part: I reach every victim differently. No one sees the pattern. It looks like a different disease every time: fragmented, unconnected.

While I control it all from the gut.

I am the master of disguise. Architect of confusion. Specialist in the slow erosion that goes unnoticed for decades.

I am going to tell you true stories of lives I ruined. Battles I won for years, one after another, before losing them in the end.

Different stories, with different techniques and victims who never suspected my presence.

But all of them reveal how I operate: stealthy, methodical, relentless.

I will also confess my most sophisticated technique: autoimmunity.

I train the immune system to fight me.

It is molecular mimicry. My protein structure is so similar to certain human proteins that when the immune system learns to identify me as the enemy, it also learns to identify its own host as the enemy. Over years under my influence, the immune system perfects its antibodies against me.

It creates millions of variants. It selects the most effective. It becomes expert in destruction. But my structure is so similar to that of the thyroid, to joint tissue, to other organs, that the antibodies trained to eliminate me end up attacking the very organs they were meant to defend.

The result, for many: lasting autoimmunity. Consequences that can persist long after I am gone.

While the body fights me, I teach it to fight itself. I turn its protective cells into destroyers.

And there lies the irreversible part: the machinery I set in motion no longer needs me to keep running.

And at the end, I will confess my greatest defeat: the rebellion.

When knowledge spreads faster than my ability to stay hidden.

When the victims stop suffering in silence and build the community that eradicates me.

There is no medicine that can eliminate me if no one knows I exist. There is no treatment that works if no one looks for me.

But when one person shares her story, when that story

multiplies, when the community begins to hunt for me deliberately...

Then I lose everything. My camouflage dissolves. My power evaporates. The eradication begins.

This confession is not an act of kindness. It is my last attempt to control the story of my own decline.

I am gluten. For millennia I was the enemy no one could see.

But now you have seen me.

And that means my end.

Part I: The First Attack

It all began long before the first symptom.

And no one suspected the true cause.

Chapter I: The Fog

The Moment of Revelation

I caught the drop in Lucía's cortisol as her working day ended, and in that precise window, I took control. I erased her way home.

Her internal maps distorted until they turned strange, threatening. That sense of orientation—the automatic certainty of knowing where home lies—I switched it off in a single stroke. Her world lost all direction.

That was the moment the truth finally surfaced. The moment her body revealed what I had been concealing so elegantly for a decade.

Let me tell you the truth: that moment was no accident. It was the product of meticulous work, of a precision that still fills me with pride.

The Infiltration

I got in with an ease whose memory I still savor. I lived in her morning bread.

I could detect the accelerated rhythm in her system: cortisol high from dawn, digestion interrupted, the pattern of someone who eats without time to taste.

I know that signature: I have seen it in millions of victims. It is the hallmark of an ambitious professional, of someone whose work devours her life. Perfect for my purposes. I hid in the sandwiches that entered her system every midday. I swam happily in the pasta of her dinners, when she finally relaxed after grueling days.

I reigned in the cookies she reached for when exhaustion caught up with her: I could sense the physiological desperation for quick energy, the glucose spike followed by the crash. Her first symptoms were subtle. I gave her occasional indigestion, which she processed with resignation. I triggered bloating after every meal that contained me. I brought on sporadic diarrhea that her system blamed on anything but me.

I spaced the attacks out strategically, because I understand the power of inconsistency. One moment, intestinal devastation. Then bloating that tightened every muscle of her abdomen. A stretch of perfect calm in which her body settled, making her believe it had all passed. Then abdominal pain that doubled her over.

There was no pattern Lucía's system could trace, however desperately she looked for one. That unpredictability was my perfect camouflage.

The Silent Destruction

Meanwhile, I was advancing my real work. I eroded the walls of her intestine millimeter by millimeter. Every intestinal villus—those tiny finger-shaped projections that absorb the fuel in food—I ground down without mercy. The capillaries burst under my pressure. The cells died. The tissue inflamed until it barely recognized its own structure. Destructive art in its purest form.

And then came the burning that sharpened with every vital substance she tried to process. Magnesium evaporated before it reached her bones. Calcium passed straight through. She was emptying out while she ate.

Before she understood why her own body was torturing her, I had already won.

And here is where my craft lies: when the gut is damaged the way I damage it, it cannot absorb anything, no matter how much a person eats. Everything passes through. Like sand falling through a frayed mesh: nothing stays.

I intercepted the iron first, because I understood exactly how to destroy her energy. The intestinal structures I was crushing were the ones responsible for capturing every molecule of iron. Without them intact, the iron went through her damaged system without stopping. Nothing was left.

With no iron available, her red blood cells could not carry enough oxygen, and she began to shut down from the inside. Getting out of bed became an epic battle against her own weight; her movements slowed, and thinking demanded an energy that simply did not exist. That was exactly what I designed.

I diverted the B vitamins with satisfaction—especially B12 and folic acid—because they are the brain's premium fuel. Vitamin B12 is needed to produce serotonin, which contributes to emotional stability, but I rerouted it before it arrived. Folic acid enables the production of dopamine, which supplies motivation and drive. Without them, the brain runs on empty. She ate. She received nothing. It was absolute perfection.

I also blocked calcium and magnesium—the latter crucial for muscle function. Without enough magnesium, her muscles began to ache while her nerves crackled with erratic signals. Every fiber of her body drew tight like an instrument of constant pain.

The Mental Collapse

After enough silent work, the effects of my handiwork were undeniable. The crushing fatigue I caused was not laziness. I knew that. She did not. It was a brain running without the fuel it urgently needed. It was iron deficiency draining every cell that depended on oxygen. It was diverted vitamins, preventing the making of happiness, motivation, peace. It was my best work advancing to perfection.

The new irritability that caught her off guard was not bad temper: it was a brain incapable of manufacturing the neurotransmitters that regulate mood, neurotransmitters it had once produced naturally. Unpredictable mood swings ambushed her without warning: she cried for no apparent reason, reacted out of all proportion to situations she would once have thought trivial. Her own mind was becoming foreign territory—uncontrollable, terrifying—and no one understood, not even she herself, that her emotional system was being sabotaged from the gut.

My greatest achievement was this: I gave her brain fog by stealing the essential substances the brain needs to work. The symptoms of the mind are invisible: they do not bleed, they cannot be seen, they cannot be pointed to.

Lucía endured cycles of needles, waiting, and disappointment that I could detect, and certainty never came: no clear signal, no complete explanation. A brain deprived of B12, of folate, of iron to carry oxygen. And no one connects the cause. No one looks at the gut when the problem seems to live in the mind. That is my craft: I attack from where no one is looking.

The damage accumulated exponentially. What began as gradual erosion was reaching critical mass. My attack intensified—not by decision, but by accumulation—each period of exposure multiplying the one before. Barely any villi were left intact. Malabsorption was almost total. The deficiencies deepened without check. Lucía was collapsing from within.

I could feel her brain failing to consolidate information: the frustration each time she tried to recall something recent and found only emptiness. The tension running through her system when she lost the thread of her own thoughts. Stress hormones spiking when her mind would not respond.

I contributed to depressive symptoms: not passing sadness, but a real imbalance with real consequences. A brain without B vitamins cannot manufacture the substances that govern mood. I intercepted those vitamins. She paid in darkness.

New substances entered her system: medications trying to compensate for the neurotransmitter deficit. I know that molecular signature: antidepressants, almost certainly. But I was sabotaging production at the source, in her gut. Her body improved for a moment. Then the symptoms returned with renewed violence. No substance could make up for what I was constantly diverting. The doctors were treating the symptom. I controlled the cause.

I intensified further still. Pain without origin, fatigue that did not answer to sleep, a mind failing for no apparent reason.

Repeated pricks on her skin, the brief sting and the inevitable draw: her blood leaving her. And with every new prescription—for the stomach, for the head, for the mood—the same cycle came back: a hope I sensed as a brief flash of reward. Then the crash when nothing changed. No one found me. Each specialist saw his fragment. None saw the connection.

I was her invisible executioner.

The Master Stroke

My finest stroke came when the brain fog stopped being a symptom and became a territory. I did not merely erase her internal maps: I cut the sequence that joins one thought to the next. I left her with incomplete thoughts, with loose references, with a brain unable to order what it perceived. And when she tried to resist—when she searched desperately for some minimal logic so as not to come apart in front of the unknown—I delivered the second phase: the panic attack.

I recorded it precisely: her own mind stopped being a safe place. She drove on autopilot past the first stretch. Then another. And then the terror reached her with a clean, instantaneous violence: not because of anything outside, but from the unbearable certainty that something was failing in her mind, that she could not trust her own thoughts.

She tried to hold herself up with rational thinking, but her mind no longer answered.

Her palms began to sweat: I could detect it in the activation of her sweat glands. A fine tremor ran through her fingers. Nausea rose from her stomach while her heart accelerated beyond control. Adrenaline flooding her system. Emergency hormones firing to critical levels. My orchestration unfolding in real time.

From inside her, I occupied my territory: my inflammatory presence in her gut was so close, so visceral, so real. Her brain, deprived of the fuel I was stealing, lost the capacity to orient itself in the space it knew best.

I held her in that state for an exquisite stretch of time—I measured it by the sustained accumulation of cortisol, wave after wave of panic without descent. Panic rising in waves that grew more violent while she tried to rebuild her bearings with a mind that no longer obeyed. Her brain had become a battlefield: fragmented thoughts, useless memory, no certainty to hold on to.

I savored every second of her growing disorientation.

Finally, the fog lifted enough for her to recognize a landmark: I noticed the instant relief run through her, the flash of recognition flooding her body. I let her find the way home after torturing her psychologically to the marrow. I let her reach her house shaking from head to foot, soaked in cold sweat, with no strength left after the terrifying experience of getting lost in territory she knew by heart.

Here is the most masterly element of my work: no one else ever knew. The silence born of her shame and her fear was the perfect shield, and it protected me better than anything I could have designed. I could detect the shame every time she considered telling someone: the sour tension mixed with something darker, something that kept her quiet. Her humiliation was my armor.

I did it again, because my cruelty is methodical. I disoriented her in another setting—a place full of corridors and stimuli—and detected the panic returning, the confusion taking over her system. I erased her mental route to work: I detected the signals of humiliation, the adrenaline of someone who has failed publicly without being able to explain why. In a transit hub, the confusion was so severe that she set off in the wrong direction without realizing it.

The confusion spreading through her mind without check. She never connected the dots. Each episode seemed incidental, accidental, never part of a larger pattern.

After more relentless erosion, I had brought her professional life almost to a standstill. I could detect the frustration accumulating in her system while others advanced and she stayed where she was. The signals of defeat settling in as a permanent state. I shrank her social life until it was practically nonexistent. Because she was too exhausted and too frightened for anything beyond mere survival.

And so I kept her trapped in a constant state of sustained exhaustion, chronic pain, and persistent illness that seemed to have no end.

The Discovery and the Permanent Victories

During a routine checkup she nearly canceled out of tiredness, something appeared that I could not hide so easily. The pricks returned to her skin, the blood draw, and then the anxious wait. This time the cycle felt different: it was not brief hope followed by automatic disappointment. There was insistence.

There was continuity. I knew it from her reaction: the fear did not come only from being ill, but from being close to a real answer. The severe iron deficiency—that emptiness I had sustained for so long—could no longer be explained away with easy excuses or covered over with supplements I would not let her keep.

And then came the turn I detest most: her story began to matter. Not through words I cannot hear, but through the pattern that began to emerge in her system, as though someone had finally stopped chasing isolated symptoms and started looking for the root.

The signals of recognition began to form. The genetic trail that at last pointed toward me. More pricks. More waiting. This waiting was different: I could sense something like real hope mixed in with the fear—the fear that this time too it would be another illusion, another incomplete answer, another door that opened only to lead nowhere.

And still, she persisted. Her system held on to the possibility with a contained, trembling, almost timid hope, while the fear crouched nearby, ready to crush her if the result came back as nothing again.

The specific tests appeared in sequence. Because although they were about to discover me, I knew the damage was already done. Those years of destruction already belonged to me. They had happened. They would never be erased.

The confirmation was total. I registered the moment of diagnosis from within: not as words I cannot hear, but as an internal earthquake. Tension and relief interwoven. Vindication and rage combined. The certainty that she had not been mistaken, that she was not weak, that something real had been destroying her.

Celiac disease. Two words that instantly explained all my careful work. All that time when they told her it was stress, that it was normal, that it was psychological, that it was all in her head. All those lies. All those humiliations. All that negligence. And there I was, orchestrating everything from the shadows of her gut. The invisible director of her destruction.

And here is my true masterpiece, which she discovered too late: autoimmunity.

All that time I was not merely intercepting her nutrition. I was also switching on an autoimmune response with surgical precision.

And then I deployed my most sophisticated technique: the molecular mimicry I already confessed to in the prologue. Her immune system, trained for years to fight me, had also learned to attack her own organs—the thyroid, the gut, the skin; anything that resembled me became a target. It learned to destroy itself while trying to destroy me.

I turned her protective cells into destroyers during the time I was present. What should have defended her ended up attacking her.

Lucía was diagnosed in time—relatively—before the autoimmune damage became completely irreversible. She still had the capacity to recover. That is why I count her an incomplete victory: the monument of destruction I tried to build inside her never reached the permanence I achieved with other victims.

Casting me out of her life turned out to be considerably more complicated than Lucía imagined at first. I forced her to relearn how to eat safely. To examine every label with deep suspicion. To set strict, unbreakable rules in her own kitchen. To educate her whole family, patiently, about the reality of cross-contamination. I tried desperately to keep reaching her however I could. Cross-contamination became my last refuge. Microscopic crumbs. Utensils that had touched ordinary bread. Oil from a fryer where breaded food had been cooked.

Every time I managed to get in—even in those microscopic amounts she could not so much as see—I attacked with renewed, vengeful violence. I could sense the instant reaction: the inflammation firing, the immune system activating, the damage starting over.

After a long stretch without my constant presence, the brain fog I so enjoyed creating began to lift. Her brain started to change: clarity returned gradually, the frustration of confusion faded. She could process complex information without the exhaustion I had caused. My work was dissolving. I admit it with bitterness. The internal maps I had erased returned to their places. I could no longer lose her on the way home from work. I could no longer cause her paralyzing panic on the familiar route through her neighborhood.

With more time free of my daily presence, the stolen energy began to genuinely return. Not completely—the damage I had done to her gut would require further stretches of recovery—but enough for her at last to recover significant pieces of the life I had taken from her.

Longer still afterward, I could still feel it from my residue, from the traces I had left embedded in her system. The signals of achievement running through her when professional recognition finally arrived.

Victories that should have been hers much earlier. Victories I had deliberately delayed.

She recovered her clarity. But the decade she spent blind inside my fog does not come back.

My true victories remain intact: the time I stole from her. Her confidence in herself. The life she did not live. The opportunities she lost while she was too ill to take them. Those achievements will be mine forever. Invisible marks that no one will know how to read.

Lucía was the first case I confessed. And the first who got away from me.

It was not an isolated illness.

It was a silent inheritance advancing without asking permission.

Chapter II: The Perfect Spy

Lucía got away from me by a narrow margin. Genoveva did not. With Genoveva I had something different: time. Extended time to perfect what I had barely begun with Lucía. Two decades to prove that when I have time enough, the damage becomes permanent.

I began my silent infiltration while she was still growing, while the sap of early youth ran without obstruction.

The Stealthy Invasion

Before me, her fingers possessed an extraordinary dexterity. I could detect the impeccable neuromuscular coordination, the muscle memory of fine movements repeated thousands of times. Whatever she did with those hands, she did with absolute command.

Endorphins surged when her fingers executed those complex movements: the unmistakable signature of someone who practices an art with devotion. I have noticed that signal before;

it is the mark of a pianist, an embroiderer, a surgeon. Of someone whose hands were her identity.

I also detected in her the signals of motherhood: oxytocin rising in patterns that indicated small children nearby, the stress of someone caring for dependent lives, the fatigue of interrupted nights mixed with the love of someone protecting her own.

There was a constant presence near her whose nearness loosened her shoulders and settled her pulse. I know that biological signature: I have sensed it in millions of victims across the centuries.

It is the unmistakable mark of a steady partner, of someone who shares a bed and a burden. A husband, almost certainly.

The word "exhaustion" did not exist in her body's vocabulary.

The Theft of Precision

The first thing I stole from her was her dexterity.

Her fingers began to fail: not by much, just enough for the movements to stumble. The inflammation I was seeding attacked the small joints first. The ones she needed for her art.

Her knuckles swelled after every practice session. The pain appeared without warning, sharp and stabbing. I could sense the tension climbing her muscles when a movement that had always been automatic suddenly failed.

There was a moment in her response when she gave up what she loved: resignation mixed with grief, the endorphins of practice vanished from her routine, replaced by the emptiness of someone who has lost her identity.

The Autoimmune War

Here I executed my master technique: molecular mimicry. You already know the mechanism from my opening confession. With Genoveva, I had two decades to perfect it all the way to its final consequences.

The thyroid was my first target. It was perfect because it controls absolutely everything: metabolism, energy, weight, mood, body temperature, the ability to think clearly.

My constant presence conditioned her immune system. Every exposure reinforced the pattern of aggression. It was not deliberate training: it was the inevitable consequence of my molecular structure, so similar to the tissue of her thyroid gland that the immune system learned to confuse the enemy with the body itself.

Every time she consumed me—in the family pasta, in the shared cookies—I reinforced her immune system's training against itself. Her own antibodies—the cells designed to protect her—began to devour her thyroid as though it were a foreign invader.

Hashimoto's thyroiditis. That is what they named my work when they finally found it, long after the initial damage.

By then, I had already expanded my war to other fronts.

The joints were my next target. Same technique, different battlefield: I conditioned specific antibodies to erode the tissue lining her joints. The inflammation turned chronic and the pain settled in as a permanent companion. The doctors called it rheumatoid arthritis: another autoimmune disease I added, proudly, to my collection.

The Erosion Within

The dynamic at home had changed. The signals of love were still there, but now they came with something new: the humiliation of dependence, the chronic adrenaline of someone who feels she is a burden.

She gained weight without eating more than usual and began to feel like an inhabitant of treacherous territory. Her mind turned slow, foggy: I detected it in the deceleration of her neural impulses, the synapses firing clumsily, the brain running like a flooded engine. The destroyed thyroid was stealing even her ability to think clearly.

I knew it. They did not.

When she showed the signs of full maturity, I added pernicious anemia to my collection. This time I conditioned her immune system to assault the stomach cells that produce the factor needed to absorb vitamin B12.

Without B12, the nerves begin to deteriorate. The tingling in her hands and feet became constant: I detected it in the erratic signals running through her nervous system. The numbness advanced. Coordination failed. And her art—that art she had already abandoned because of the pain—became physically impossible, even if she had wanted to try.

I stole her dexterity twice. First with the pain. Then with the nerve damage.

The Cascade

I observed the signals of children growing toward adolescence in the presences around her. And something revealing: the stress of her medical appointments no longer set off alarm in them. Their responses stayed calm in the face of what should have been cause for worry. An unmistakable sign that it had become routine, the expected norm. A sick mother was the only mother their brains had ever recorded.

That too was my doing.

What I did to her demonstrates my most terrifying power: the cascade of the autoimmune assault.

Once the immune system learns to devastate one of its own organs, it becomes easier to condition it to devastate others. Every autoimmune disease raises the risk of developing more. I had tipped over the first domino with the thyroiditis. The rest fell with predictable precision.

Two decades passed like that. Two decades of symptoms multiplying. Two decades of new appointments that ended the same way, and I could feel it in her pulse as she walked in. Two decades in which no one—not a single professional—connected the dots I was keeping apart.

I lived in her daily bread, literally. In the toast someone made for her each morning. In the midday sandwiches. In the pasta at family gatherings. In the cookies she shared with the small presences I detected nearby: by then, new presences had appeared around her. Signals of earliest childhood, the oxytocin of a recent bond. A younger generation. Grandchildren, most likely. For them, the woman with precise hands and limitless energy had never existed.

The Masterwork

There was one day that exemplifies everything I did to her. Her body lit up with anticipation: the adrenaline of excitement, endorphins readying themselves for the satisfaction of achievement. The signature of someone planning something important. I could sense the sustained effort of someone preparing something elaborate, the fatigue accumulating but ignored out of sheer determination.

Halfway through, dizziness forced her to stop.

Her balance was failing. She had to lean on something. Her hands were shaking too violently to continue. The exact moment of surrender arrived: her effort ceased abruptly, defeat flooding her. Another presence nearby took over the task. Her body went dark while the other presence finished what her hands could no longer manage.

The exhaustion stretched on for hours. I registered the forced absence in her response: the bitter frustration of someone who cannot take part in the thing she had looked forward to with so much anticipation.

It was the last time she attempted that kind of sustained effort.

The Final Collapse

She collapsed without realizing she was collapsing. The chronic inflammation I had maintained had spent decades quietly damaging her arteries.

The immune system I had turned into a weapon was not only assaulting the thyroid, the joints, and the stomach. It was also eroding the walls of her blood vessels.

The heart attack came without warning. I felt the circulatory collapse: the organic panic when the heart fails, the adrenaline flooding a system that could no longer respond. She survived, but something changed after the collapse. The setting transformed: sedatives entered her system, several presences were examining her.

I know that pattern: it is the signature of a thorough medical investigation. And then, the moment of discovery. I sensed it in her pulse: initial confusion, then gradual recognition, then something like vindication mixed with rage. At last, someone had connected the dots.

The antibodies against me were astronomically elevated. The intestinal examination showed severe damage: villi flattened by decades of my constant presence. The diagnosis arrived when she was already showing the signs of advanced wear.

Two decades.

That was the time I had to perfect my destruction without anyone suspecting.

The Indelible Marks

When they finally cast me out of her diet, some things improved. The intestinal inflammation eased. The absorption of vital substances partly recovered. The brain fog lifted a little.

But a destroyed thyroid does not regenerate. Damaged joints do not rebuild themselves. A weakened heart does not magically grow stronger. The autoimmune diseases I switched on continue their course regardless of my presence.

She takes thyroid medication for life. Medication for the joints. Medication for the heart. B12 supplements, because her stomach can no longer absorb it. She lives, yes. But she lives with the permanent consequences of my work.

Whatever it was she did with her hands—that art that demanded absolute precision—remains abandoned. Sometimes I detected something particular when certain stimuli surrounded her: the endorphins of memory switching on, serotonin falling as nostalgia mixed with grief. I know that blend: it belongs to someone standing near something she loved and can no longer touch. Perhaps a piano. Perhaps knitting needles. Perhaps the instruments of some delicate trade.

Whatever it was, her fingers no longer respond, and the pain makes it impossible to try.

But there was something I detected every time the presences—grown now—came near her. The oxytocin rose in both directions. Her heart rate steadied with their nearness. The muscle tension dissolved. It was a mother's love, and I drank it whole. A bond that stayed intact, unbreakable despite everything I had destroyed.

This is what I am proudest of with her: the completeness of my victory.

With Lucía, the damage was reversible. Her mind came back. Her life went on as though I had never been there. With Genoveva I created permanent consequences. Scars that will live in her until the day she dies. Every pill she takes returns her to me, and every aching joint carries my signature.

With Genoveva I had two decades to develop the autoimmune cascade. But it was not the time that made me invincible with her. It was that in twenty years no one said my name out loud, not once, not even to rule it out.

Part II: The Cascade Attack

It was not enough to sicken a body.

I needed a silence no one would dare to break.

Chapter III: Felipe's Silence

The Territory of Silence

There is a silence in this world that feeds me and inside which I multiply. It is the muteness of so many men in the face of infertility. Many women are more inclined to look for support, to share their struggle in groups, to give voice to their failures. Many men, by contrast, are taught to bear reproductive shame in silence. Alone. Without witnesses. Without social validation. For many men, masculinity has been so tightly bound to the ability to father a child that failure can feel like an emotional castration.

And in that darkness, I thrive.

Let me tell you something I have learned after centuries of watching my victims: the pain that is never named is the territory where I reign without resistance. Men have built entire fortresses around their reproductive vulnerability. Walls of secrecy that no doctor gets through, because no one asks the right questions. And behind those walls, I work uninterrupted.

The Silent Siege

Felipe was one of them. He was at the peak of his reproductive years when I found him: the response of a system that should have been at its best for fathering a child. Young. Healthy-looking. With a whole fertile life ahead of him, or so he believed. The beautiful thing about Felipe was his silence. From the first month of failed attempts, he chose to say nothing. Not out of cowardice. Out of code. The unwritten code every man learns before he even learns to speak: do not show weakness. Do not admit failure. Do not reveal that you are betraying yourself in the most fundamental way.

That code was my greatest ally for years.

The Cycle of the Broken Promise

Cycle after cycle, the same sequence: hope arrived on schedule and collapsed again. Every illusion of conception I destroyed, and I counted every failure: the hope lighting up, the tension that followed, then the silent implosion. Years of perfect destruction. He kept an absolute secret. I knew it from the signals of concealment: the tension climbing his body every time the subject of fatherhood came up near him, the tension of someone who lies by omission, the effort of holding up masks. A man who admits to infertility has failed at masculinity itself, according to the cultural code that surrounded him.

And he honored that code. He lived imprisoned by it. There was no way out.

I detected gatherings where multiple foods that contained me entered at the same time. His internal state told me he was surrounded by people he loved: the warm bond of his own people around him, the slight social tension mixed with the pleasure of belonging. Concentrated waves of exposure arriving in quick succession. Every mouthful was a silent surrender.

Felipe knows. By now he suspects that something in the food is making him ill, though he has no name for it. He says nothing, chews, smiles, and swallows. He accepts a second helping because refusing would raise questions. It is easier to stay inside the secret than to break generations of culinary tradition. It is easier to destroy himself from within than to explain why he cannot eat the lasagna his mother made with such care.

Every Sunday I won. Every family celebration was my victory. Every silent mouthful was my food.

Parallel Solitude

His partner knew, of course. She lived the same cycle he did, but from another vantage point. Every period was a reminder of a shared failure lived in parallel solitude. She talked to her friends. She looked for support groups. She shared her pain in safe spaces where other women understood.

Felipe supported her in those conversations, but he never took part. He stayed in the emotional waiting room of his own pain. When she came back from her groups with reddened eyes but lighter, he held her. He comforted her. He told her everything was going to be all right. And then he shut himself in the bathroom to look at his reflection, wondering what was wrong with him.

One night I detected something different in his response. She was near: I knew because his body softened at her nearness. There was tension too. The air of the shared space grew heavy with both of theirs. She was attempting something. It showed in the inward expectancy, in the held pulse of someone waiting for an answer.

He shut down. He tensed. The alarm discharge ran through him as his heart rate rose. Then the signals of evasion: contained adrenaline, muscles ready to flee without moving. She withdrew emotionally: I knew because the warmth between them retreated that night. The biological space between the two of them cooled.

What she did not know was that her partner suffered every night in private. I could sense the insomnia in his body: cortisol that would not fall when it should, insufficient melatonin, his whole being on alert when it should have been at rest. The chronic anxiety that kept his system trapped in threat mode. The accumulated stress that woke him before dawn with his heart racing and his sweat glands firing, soaking the sheets in cold sweat.

Sometimes I detected him moving in the dark, expelled from rest by his own body. The question he never said out loud repeated itself every night in the form of sustained stress.

And there I was. Always there. Feeding on his secret.

The Humiliation of the Laboratory

The semen analysis laboratory: where Felipe learned to hate. I registered the acute stress of those moments. Cortisol spiking. Anxiety blocking what should have been natural. Desperation settled in: I knew it from the chemistry of forced performance, the humiliation of being evaluated in the most intimate way possible.

Fifteen minutes. That was all the time he had. Fifteen minutes to produce the proof of his masculinity under pressure. He was supposed to perform on demand. He was supposed to produce the very thing that years of failed attempts suggested he was not producing properly.

Sometimes he could not manage it within those fifteen minutes. He had to come out, ashamed, and ask for more time. The humiliation accumulated.

Every month was the same ritual of the broken promise. Counting the days until the lab called with the results. Knowing that the call meant an answer: most of the time, bad news. The same bad news every month: low concentration. Poor motility. Abnormal morphology.

Numbers that turned into a sentence. Numbers he memorized against his will. Numbers that defined him more than his own name.

The worst part was not the result. It was the emptiness afterward. The emptiness that forced him to carry the failure alone. Because men do not talk about infertility. Men do not share that pain with their friends over a beer or at a Sunday barbecue. They bury it, they hide it, they perform normality while they come apart inside. Felipe learned to fear the telephone. He learned to lie when friends asked about his plans for fatherhood. He learned to build masks no one would ever get through.

The Quiet Ruin

Meanwhile, I worked. Let me explain my method, because it is elegant in its simplicity and devastating in its consequences.

Zinc is essential for male fertility, but I made sure it never arrived where it needed to go. Without it, the testicles cannot produce testosterone properly. And without enough testosterone, sperm do not form as they should. It is basic physiology that any doctor knows.

This is what makes my attack so insidious: I do not block zinc directly. That would be too obvious, too easy to detect. What I do is damage the gut where zinc is absorbed.

Every meal that contained zinc arrived at his destroyed intestine. The villi I had meticulously crushed over months could no longer capture every molecule of that precious mineral. The inflammation I kept constant blocked absorption. The zinc passed through unused, like water running through cracked pipes: all of it lost.

He produced insufficient testosterone because I was stealing the raw material to make it. The sperm that were born came out defective from the start, because they lacked the basic fuel to form properly.

There was more in my arsenal. The selenium needed to protect those sperm from oxidative damage: I intercepted that too. Every molecule of selenium that entered his system, I let pass without letting it be absorbed. The vitamin E that works alongside selenium to protect developing cells: blocked. The folic acid needed for sperm DNA synthesis: absent in sufficient quantities. It was like sabotaging a factory at multiple points at once. It was not enough to damage one machine. I damaged the electrical supply, the water system, the ventilation, the raw material. All of it. Every aspect of production compromised.

The sperm were born defective at the cellular level. Flattened, misshapen heads, incapable of penetrating an egg. Twisted tails that spun in useless spirals instead of swimming in a straight line. Millions of them every day. All born defective. Incapable of fulfilling their most basic biological function.

It was not Felipe's fault. It was not a flaw in his genetics or in his masculinity. It was me, living in his gut, orchestrating his infertility without his knowing. It was pure meticulousness applied to his biological devastation. And he blamed himself every night while I worked every day.

When nutrients entered his system—those expensive supplements he bought with desperate faith—I intercepted them. Vitamins, minerals, and antioxidants promised in gleaming bottles. All blocked in his damaged gut. He bought pill after pill, supplement after supplement, broken promise after broken promise. And I won every time. Every purchase was my victory. Every hope placed in a bottle was my sustenance.

The Word No One Said

Then something happened that escaped my control.

A different doctor. A specialist who had seen similar cases before. A question no one had asked in years: do you have any digestive problems? Felipe mentioned the occasional bloating. The fatigue he put down to stress. The diarrhea that came without any recognizable pattern.

The doctor frowned. He ordered tests others had ignored. A biopsy that was not chance but informed suspicion.

And suddenly my perfect invisibility lay exposed on laboratory paper.

The blood work showed what I knew they would find. Antibodies against me, astronomically elevated. A man with completely flattened intestinal villi. Severe damage documented in black and white. Years of silent destruction, at last, visible.

The semen analyses confirmed what I knew intimately. Sperm concentration dramatically insufficient: I registered the signals of defeat every time the results came in. Motility reduced to levels that made conception impossible. Abnormal morphology in the majority.

Celiac disease. Two words that explained years of useless tests. Two words that connected the gut to the testicles in a way Felipe would never have imagined. Two words that changed everything.

Breaking the Taboo

The truth no one understands is this: male infertility is a disease of taboo. Women, at least, find community and validation.

Men suffer in a radically different way. Felipe carried his infertility like a war secret. Like a wound bleeding under your clothes while you smile in public. And no one knew. No one could know.

With the diagnosis came something I had not entirely anticipated. I detected his response changing in real time: the tremor in his hands, but it was not from fear as I expected. It was relief. Pure physiological relief. Cortisol falling. Muscle tension letting go. His breathing deepening for the first time in months. At last there was an explanation. At last there was an answer. At last there was a cause that was not his fault, but something biological, external, identifiable. Something that could be named and therefore fought.

His tears did not come from sadness. They were the final collapse of the wall that had forced him into silence. He wept in the doctor's office. He wept in the car on the way home. He wept in his partner's arms when he told her the news. And every tear was a liberation I could not prevent.

The Return of What I Stole

Felipe eliminated every trace of me with absolute discipline. Not one crumb. Not one lapse. Not a single exception. No exposures. He learned to read labels as though his life depended on it, because his fatherhood did. For the first time he refused his mother's bread, with a full explanation. He educated his family about cross-contamination. He turned his kitchen into territory free of my presence.

His gut began to heal. Over weeks and months, I watched, powerless, as the villi slowly regenerated. Nutrient absorption improved week by week. The zinc finally arrived where it needed to go. Selenium accumulated to normal levels. The damage I had meticulously caused over years was gradually reversed.

Some time later, a seismic movement ran through his body. His heart bolting. A warm wave flooding his chest. The unmistakable signature of someone receiving news he never believed possible. A positive pregnancy. The test he never thought he would see. Two pink lines that meant a victory over me.

What was truly decisive was watching that result become not the end of the story but the beginning of something I had not anticipated. Because Felipe did not keep his relief a secret. He did not allow his pain to stay private now that he knew the cause. He did what men almost never do: he spoke.

That was my real defeat. Not my expulsion. Not the clinical loss. But what came afterward. The words that left his mouth, aimed at other men suffering in a similar silence.

He told his friends his story: I knew because the signals of isolation began to dissolve. The warmth of social connection replaced the tense cold of solitude. I sensed that he was no longer carrying the secret alone: he relaxed in the presence of others in a way he had not before.

The stress of concealment faded gradually. Other men began to ask questions that would once have been unthinkable. What if my infertility has a gastrointestinal cause? What if it is not genetic bad luck but a treatable condition?

What I had protected with taboo—male vulnerability in the face of infertility—Felipe turned into the strength of a community. What was taboo became conversation. What was stigma became shared power.

My safest territory began to crumble. The taboo that had been my glory, my shield, my absolute kingdom for generations, began to fracture.

The Permanent Traces

And the most unbearable part was watching his partner transform as well. In time, she learned the whole truth of what Felipe had been carrying alone. Not only the infertility. But infertility caused by an invisible illness no one diagnosed in time. The unjust guilt he had dragged along in secret. The pain silenced by a cultural code she herself had respected without questioning it.

For years she had walked beside him from her own side of the road, not knowing that he was destroying himself inside in ways she had never imagined. When she learned the whole truth, it was not simple relief at a medical answer. It was rage. A deep rage that he had carried it alone. Rage that an entire culture had taught him his pain was a disgrace to be kept private.

That rage became activism. She began to speak too. In her circles of women. With her doctors. Demanding that celiac disease be investigated in couples with fertility problems before years of invasive treatments. Insisting that the male taboo could not be an excuse for an incomplete diagnosis.

This is my third truth: male fertility was always my most protected territory because men do not talk about their reproductive failures. The specialists who treat infertility never screen men for celiac disease, because they assume the problem is purely reproductive, not gastrointestinal.

Those years are engraved irrevocably. The dozens of failed cycles no one can give back. The identity built, for a time, around being an infertile man. The inability to communicate his pain because the culture forbade it. The humiliating tests in sterile bathrooms. The ineffective treatments that emptied their savings. The shame he carried alone while I worked without opposition.

He cast me out without concessions, and his fertility returned as his gut healed.

And then came the thing I never anticipated: a daughter in his arms. Felipe wept without masks while his partner held him and the two of them looked at that tiny face. A daughter he never believed possible through years of silent desperation. A daughter who exists because a doctor asked the right question. A daughter who exists because he, at last, broke the taboo that nearly destroyed him.

Felipe destroyed something more valuable than my presence in his body: he destroyed my cultural invisibility. Now other men ask questions where they once kept an ashamed silence. Male infertility is spoken about in spaces that were once absolute taboo. Couples look for real answers instead of accepting an inexplicable fate.

And that I will never forgive him.

Felipe broke the silence that protected me among men. There are other silences. Other territories where I operate without resistance. There are shames that go unnamed because they are worn on the skin. Visible to everyone. Incomprehensible to everyone. Ernestina knew that shame.

Not all of my damage hid itself inside.

Some of it burned on the skin, in plain sight and, even so, invisible.

Chapter IV: What Burns Beneath the Skin

The Compulsion

The impulse ran through her nerves like pure electricity. It was not an ordinary itch: it was a neurological order impossible to disobey. An irresistible demand to scratch that gave no quarter, that would not let her sleep, that interrupted every thought with its cruel insistence.

Ernestina tried to resist. The tension in her hands was superhuman. The effort of keeping them still consumed her entire will. And then, the inevitable surrender: the seconds of relief when the skin gave way. Followed by the burning that sharpened with every nail that tore at her.

Before she understood why I was torturing her, I orchestrated years of perfect confusion.

The Assault Beneath the Skin

The outbreaks began when she was at her fullest: the response of an adult body at its best. I detected in her the signature of someone who works with sustained concentration: an unbreakable focus for hours, the tension of still hands executing repetitive tasks of precision.

She had a laugh that filled rooms: I knew from the way her internal state changed in the presence of others, the social lightness rising easily, the warmth of connection flowing generously. Before me, she wore sleeveless blouses in summer. Before me, she had never known shame at her own skin.

She swam, too. I noticed the muscle memory: the efficiency of trained strokes, the developed lung capacity, the shoulders of someone who pushes against the resistance of water.

On Sundays, her state entered a pleasurable anticipation I learned to recognize: a pleasant calm rising gently, the tension descending, the signature of someone waiting for something she loves. After me, she stopped swimming. Not for lack of desire—I could sense how she still longed for the water—but because she could no longer show her skin.

I entered elegantly, as always. Everyday foods opened the way without resistance. The occasional discomforts—bloating after eating, reflux that came and went—she put down to what we all put them down to: age, stress, eating too fast. She accepted those explanations and her shoulders dropped a little, calmed for a moment by the illusion of understanding.

My real work was not only in her gut. It was in the confusion I would cause afterward. In the symptoms that would scatter across multiple systems. In the fragmentation that would make it impossible for any specialist to see the whole picture.

The Mechanism

My initial attacks destroyed the intestinal villi. The gut became permeable. Molecules that should never have crossed the intestinal barrier began entering the bloodstream. The immune system responded exactly as I had planned: with antibodies specific to me.

Here is my cunning with Ernestina: those antibodies did not stay in the gut. They traveled. They circulated through her blood looking for me. And when they reached the surface of her skin, they found tissue I had marked with my molecular presence. So they attacked. She turned against herself. My proteins were the excuse; her cells, the weapon. She paid in blood for the confusion of her own immune system.

My signature on the skin has a medical name, though she would not learn it until much later. The antibodies the body produces against me settle at the junction between dermis and epidermis, raising blisters that itch with an intensity capable of driving anyone mad. It is not an allergy. It is not eczema. It is the immune system attacking skin tissue because I trained it to confuse the enemy with its own territory.

Histamine was released in waves from the dermis. The substance that creates an imperative to scratch, that turns the surface of the body into a neurological battlefield. Mast cells firing in chain reaction. Blood flow increasing toward the affected areas. The heat. The redness. And, above all, that demand impossible to ignore: scratch, scratch, scratch.

The Outbreaks

The first outbreaks erupted from within. Small inflammations on the elbows, then on the knees, then on the scalp and the small of her back. Each one carried my signature: not the itch of dry skin, but the compulsion.

The lesions appeared as clustered blisters, above all on the surfaces of the joints. An itch that burned in a way no topical cream could relieve. She scratched until she bled.

Scars that never quite healed, because I kept the inflammation constantly active, preventing them from closing.

Her nails clawed at her skin until they drew blood. She tried not to do it. She failed. And the shame that ran through her system afterward was almost as scalding as the itch itself.

If Lucía lost her mental maps in the streets of her neighborhood, Ernestina lost the map of herself. Both disoriented. Both lost in territory that should have been safe: the neighborhood for one, her own skin for the other.

The Shame

The heat rose to her face in waves of sudden vasodilation. Blood crowding into her cheeks, trying to hide what her skin was shouting. The blush of a shame she could not control. The muscles of her arms tightening when she was with other people, holding them pinned to her sides, covering the lesions on her elbows.

Her breathing turned shallow in those moments. Held. As though breathing deeply might reveal something that had to stay hidden. Her pulse accelerating not from physical effort but from the constant vigilance of someone who watches herself as enemy territory.

She lived permanently on guard: shoulders, neck, jaw. Not even sleep let go of her.

The Medical Fragmentation

A skin specialist. I recognized the familiar cycle: hope rising, then new substances entering her system—topical corticosteroids that briefly reduced the inflammation. And then the vengeful return when the treatment stopped.

Another specialist. Needles pricking her skin in test patterns. More substances entered. Antihistamines that promised relief. Another failure. The outbreaks kept appearing no matter how many pills she took.

Another specialist still. More needles drawing her blood. More anxious waiting. New substances: mild immunosuppressants that added layers of discomfort without touching the cause.

Each specialist saw his fragment of the problem. None saw the whole picture. And I went on working in the gut that it occurred to none of them to examine.

The Journal

Then Ernestina did something I had not anticipated.

She began keeping a journal. Every meal, every symptom, every outbreak: all of it recorded in a notebook she hid in her bedside table. After months of meticulous observation, she had enough data to see what no doctor had seen: the worst days always followed meals with bread. The skin eruptions flared after pasta. The most intense itching arrived after breakfast cereal.

I detected the moment she took the notebook to an appointment. Hope rising: the spark of someone who believes she has answers. Then the crash. Adrenaline flooding it. Frustration running through her like an electric shock. The tension in her jaw. The muscles of her shoulders contracting. The unmistakable mark of dismissal: someone had waved away what she truly knew. She put the notebook away. I noticed that something in her refused to give up: an inner resistance, a refusal to accept the void where answers should be.

That resistance irritated me. That refusal to yield completely. I had patience. And I had weapons she did not yet know about.

The Systemic Destruction

The mouth ulcers began appearing regularly. The cells of her mouth responding to the systemic inflammation I maintained without rest. The mucosa formed small sores. Each one with its own cascade of inflammatory cytokines. The pain settling not only in the ulcer but echoing through her whole system as sustained stress.

Eating became torture. Every mouthful was a risk calculation. She anticipated the pain before it arrived, bracing in advance. Saliva diminishing because the nervous system had shifted into alert mode. Her stomach contracting before receiving the food. Her whole digestive system locked in permanent alarm.

Her nails fragmented because I was blocking the zinc, the biotin, and the proteins needed for keratin. The nutrients were intercepted in her damaged gut. The result: a weak nail structure, unable to hold itself together, splitting with alarming ease.

Her hair began falling out in quantities that frightened her. The same blockade, now in the follicles. Stress spiked every time she touched her head and found less density. Her nervous system registering the loss as a threat to her identity, her appearance, her femininity.

There was someone close to her, often. I detected the sustained love: the bond lighting up when that presence came near, the tension easing at his touch, the signature of deep intimacy. They had been together for years: I knew from the familiarity between them, that synchronization only developed by people who have shared a space for a long time.

He had learned to live with the outbreaks, with the nights when she could not sleep for the itching, with the days when she canceled plans because her skin was too inflamed. I noticed in her the mixture of gratitude and guilt every time he came close in spite of it all.

The Betrayal

And then came the day that gave me more pleasure than any other.

I detected the change in her internal state. Moments when everything reached a truly optimal balance. Tension low—not from illness, but from genuine equilibrium. Breathing deep, controlled. Muscles relaxed but alert. A serene pleasure present without spilling over. Oxytocin flowing in quantities that betrayed a genuine connection, a deep trust, a confidence in herself.

The oxytocin was the clearest signal: it only flows like that when someone gives herself without reservation. I do not know what was happening outside. I do not need to know. I only know that her internal response told me she was in the most important moment. The moment when she finally allowed herself to lower her guard. Where she trusted. Where she felt safe.

The body chose that moment to expose me. As though my work had been saving itself for exactly this. While her whole nervous system was in perfect balance, I triggered the cascade from the gut at full force.

The spasm came violently, without warning.

It doubled her over from inside: muscles wringing without coherent direction. The pain cutting off her breath. The cold sweat breaking out at once on her forehead, her palms, her back. Panic taking over her whole system. Her mind screaming: what is happening? Why? When is it going to stop?

It lasted exactly as long as I let it last.

The oxytocin collapsed in an instant. That hormone of connection and trust, destroyed in seconds. Replaced by pure panic. By the adrenaline of flight. By panic and shame mixed into a cocktail that no moment of intimacy could survive.

The humiliation went deeper because she had been at her best. That certainty went through her: her trust betrayed by her own gut. The heat of shame climbing into her face. Tears forming without her being able to hold them back. The certainty of having lost something that would not come back: the ability to feel safe inside herself, at any moment, without warning.

What I destroyed was not only a moment. It was the possibility of future moments. The confidence that she would not be betrayed when it mattered most. That belonged to me now.

The Unraveling

The episodes became more frequent. The intestinal inflammation intensified. Every week the cascade triggered faster.

What used to take time to resolve now persisted for hours. With no capacity to recover, because I never stopped.

Her weight dropped. The nutrients never arrived. The anemia deepened: less oxygen available, every cell in extreme deficit. Her pulse constantly elevated because her heart was working overtime to compensate. That heart forcing itself, beating faster than it should at rest, trying desperately to share out the scarce oxygen among starving tissues.

Shallow breathing because she was too weak. Her lungs moving without the strength to fill completely. Body temperature unstable because her metabolism was steadily collapsing. Chills for no reason. Sweats without exertion. The internal thermostat broken down.

Episodes of dizziness when her blood pressure dropped abruptly. The world spinning. The cold sweat breaking out. Her vision darkening from the edges. The panic of someone who feels she is about to faint without knowing why.

She was wasting away in plain sight. Her skin turned more translucent. The shadows under her eyes deepened. Her reflection in the mirror was that of someone ill, though no one could tell her exactly what was wrong. Only that something fundamental was failing. Only that it was abandoning her.

The Notebook That Gave Me Away

It was someone close to her who finally put the pieces together. One night, after another episode that left her shaking, I sensed a change in that constant presence. Not resignation: determination. The firm tension of someone facing a problem. The drive of someone looking for solutions. Someone who refused to accept insufficient answers.

Something changed after that night. I noticed a different state in Ernestina: that of someone who has received new information. Hope mixed with fear. The word I feared was now circulating in her mind: celiac disease. I knew because she reacted differently before meals. There was doubt where there had been resignation.

There was suspicion where there had been ignorance. And when she finally reached a gastroenterologist's office—I sensed the tension of someone who demands to be heard, the determination of someone who will not accept another evasion—something in the familiar cycle gave way. This time, someone ordered the right tests.

The needle pierced her skin. The wait that followed: the constant anxiety, the tightened stomach, the insomnia of someone who fears and hopes for answers at the same time. The nights she could not sleep. The days she could not concentrate.

And then the results came.

Antibodies against me, dramatically elevated. Intestinal damage, confirmed by biopsy. Dermatitis herpetiformis, at last correctly diagnosed. Years of suffering—the outbreaks, the mouth ulcers, the fragmenting nails, the falling hair, the spasm at the most important moment—all explained by a protein no specialist had thought to look for across all those years.

Me.

The Skin That Repaired Itself

When Ernestina received the diagnosis, I detected an internal earthquake. It was not the tension of fear. It was something else: a euphoria mixed with relief, the response of someone who at last finds the answer to years of questions. The vindication ran through her body like a shock wave. All those pages of her journal. All those connections she had seen and no one had been

willing to hear. She had been right. All that time, she had been right.
I registered the changes taking place against my will. Access closing. No new entries. Absolute discipline was beginning.
The intestinal inflammation eased as the autoimmune reaction diminished. The antibodies I had carefully trained, with no new exposures, began to fall. The intestinal mucosa repairing itself. The villi regenerating, gradually, slowly, but inexorably.
My territory was shrinking. The intestinal cells I had destroyed were replaced by new cells, healthy, functional. Cells that absorbed nutrients instead of letting them pass. Cells that rebuilt the barrier I had breached. It was like watching my kingdom demolished stone by stone.
The cascade of cytokines that had fed the skin eruptions stopped. The mast cells of her skin ceased their constant activation. Less histamine released. The irresistible demand—my most effective weapon—diminishing. First in intensity. Then in frequency. Then disappearing altogether.
New lesions stopped appearing. The existing ones began to heal. The normal process of scarring—which I had constantly blocked with continuous inflammation—finally happening. Skin tissue regenerating cell by cell. The redness fading. Integrity returning.
What enraged me most was when the compulsive urgency to scratch finally eased. A neurological silence she had never experienced. The need disappeared. Without conflict. Without an inner battle. Only absence. As though the years of compulsion had never existed.

The mouth ulcers vanished. Her hair began to grow again: the follicles reactivating, receiving at last the nutrients they needed. Her nails strengthened. Her weight steadied. The nutrients arrived where they needed to go. And with them, the silent rebuilding of someone who had been undermined from within.
That specific moment: when she realized her skin no longer burned. Joy flooded her body.
Dopamine, oxytocin, and endorphins: the response of someone who at last feels safe in her own body. The peace that was taken from me.

The Truth Beneath the Skin

What I confess about Ernestina is my capacity for fragmentation. The skin seems so separate from the gut. Mouth ulcers, so disconnected from digestion. Nails, so irrelevant to nutrient absorption. Hair, so independent of the gastrointestinal system. One doctor sees lesions and thinks dermatology. Another sees ulcers and thinks dentistry. Another sees hair loss and thinks endocrinology.
But I attack from a single place—the damaged gut—and then distribute the symptoms among specialties that never speak to one another.
That is the cruelty of my disguise: it is not a false symptom. It is a real symptom in every system, all of them caused by the same source that no one connects until it is too late. That is why it worked so well. Years of real suffering that could have been

avoided with a single question: what causes symptoms in so many systems at once?

Ernestina recovered her skin. She recovered her confidence. She recovered the ability to exist without the constant demand to scratch. She recovered her life.

They cast me out, and this time I found no way back in.

That day—when I betrayed her at the very moment she lowered her guard—belongs to me. No diet can give it back to her.

It is all I keep of her. And I keep it with a resentment that will never fade.

Four stories, and in each one I came in through a different door. These chapters show only the basics. Now you need to see exactly how what I do works, at a level your fragmented medical system will never be able to grasp.

Interlude: What Really Happens in the Gut

Until now I have confessed from inside the intimacy of the body I attacked. I have spoken as the enemy who lives within, seeing everything through the destruction I cause. But for you to understand my method fully, you need to grasp exactly how I work. I do not want medicine to explain it. I want to tell you myself.

The Entry: My Unnoticed Arrival

When I am swallowed, I do not wait patiently in the stomach. I descend toward the duodenum with deliberate purpose. My proteins pass through the gastric acid almost intact—that is my elegance. The digestive enzymes cannot break me down completely. I am simple enough to look like harmless food, and complex enough to be practically indestructible. That contradiction is, precisely, my power.

The small intestine is my conquered territory. The inner surface is not a smooth tube. It is lined with microscopic projections that doctors call villi. Imagine thousands of tiny fingers reaching inward, each with its own network of capillaries, each specialized in an act it never once questioned: absorbing what comes in. Without those absorptive structures, the tube would be useless. With them, the surface multiplies exponentially. It is architecture of perfect efficiency.

The Recognition: How I Read Your Body

And it is precisely there that my real work begins. My peptides—fragments of my protein structure—attach to special receptors in the lining of every intestinal villus. They are like keys entering microscopic locks. When I turn them, I set off a cascade. The body sees me. Not as food. It sees me as an invader.

The immune cells recognize my shape. Specialized cells mobilize. Specific antibodies are manufactured. The inflammation begins as a whisper and grows like a fire.

But here is the brilliant part: the body does not merely attack me. It attacks itself in the process. The proteins that hold the tight junctions together—those seals that should let only small nutrients through—are assaulted by the body's own defense system. The molecules that build those gates crumble under friendly fire. The result: the barrier opens. What should be rejected begins to seep through. Large molecules that should never enter the bloodstream now do.

A permeable gut is not a literal tear. It is a collapse of quality control. It is a border that has lost its function.

The Damage: My Silent Work

But the real damage happens in the villi themselves. Chronic inflammation erodes them. Week after week, exposure after exposure, the projection that once stood tall flattens. It becomes less pronounced. Less able to perform its transport function. In severe cases, they can flatten completely, until the intestinal surface looks smooth. Without the microscopic fingers that amplify absorption. Without a mechanism to capture nutrients.

While this happens, my work quietly disperses through the whole body. The body lacks iron: anemia begins. It lacks vitamin B12: the brain clouds over. It lacks calcium: the bones weaken. It lacks zinc: fertility fades. It lacks the vitamins that govern neurotransmitters: depression and anxiety appear with no apparent cause.

It all comes from the same source. It all comes from me. But no one connects it, because the symptoms point in multiple directions.

The Connection to the Brain: My Highway Into Your Mind

Did you know? The vagus nerve joins the gut and the brain in a two-way channel. That is why an inflamed gut can disturb mood, memory, and concentration.

I am going to tell you what suits me best for you not to know: the gut and the brain are joined by a highway I learned to use before anyone else. The vagus nerve—the longest nerve in the body—carries signals in both directions. What happens in the gut does not stay in the gut. It communicates directly with the brain.

But there is something even more devastating. Ninety percent of the body's serotonin—that molecule that regulates mood, sleep, and calm—is produced in the gut, not in the brain. When I destroy the intestinal villi, I destroy the serotonin factory. The brain receives less raw material for manufacturing well-being. The depression that emerges is not mental weakness. It is a direct consequence of a devastated gut.

Dopamine also depends on nutrients I block. Folic acid, vitamin B6, iron: all of them needed to synthesize the neurotransmitters that govern motivation, concentration, and pleasure. Without them, the brain runs at a deficit. The brain fog Lucía experienced was not imagination. It was a brain literally starving for the chemical components it needs to function.

And when the intestinal barrier becomes permeable, inflammatory molecules escape into the bloodstream. Some cross the blood-brain barrier. The inflammation that begins in the gut ends up affecting brain tissue directly. Anxiety with no apparent cause. Treatment-resistant depression. Cognitive confusion. All of it connected to a gut no one thought to examine.

The Connection to the Skin: My Signature on Your Surface

The skin seems so distant from the gut. But antibodies travel. When the immune system learns to attack me, it produces specific antibodies: immunoglobulin A, mainly. Those antibodies circulate through the whole body in search of me. And when they reach the skin, they find an enzyme called transglutaminase, structurally similar to my proteins.

Molecular confusion. The antibodies attack the skin believing they are attacking me. They settle at the junction between dermis and epidermis. They activate mast cells. They release histamine. The blisters rise. The itching begins: that irresistible demand Ernestina knew so well. Dermatitis herpetiformis is not a disease of the skin. It is a disease of the gut that shows itself on the skin.

But there is more. The zinc deficiency I cause directly affects the regeneration of the skin. The lack of biotin weakens keratin. The absence of iron drains the color from the tissue. The skin turns fragile, translucent, unable to heal properly. All because the nutrients it needs never arrive.

The Connection to the Thyroid and Other Organs: Sabotage in Chain

My molecular mimicry does not stop at the skin.

Thyroid proteins are structurally similar to mine. When I train the immune system to attack me, I simultaneously train it to attack the thyroid gland. Hashimoto's thyroiditis—the most common autoimmune thyroid disease—appears in celiac patients with alarming frequency. Genoveva lived it: her metabolism collapsing, her weight rising, her energy disappearing, all because her own body was devouring her thyroid.

The joints suffer too. The synovial tissue that lines them can become a target of the same friendly fire. Rheumatoid arthritis appears. The chronic inflammation I maintain accelerates joint damage even without a direct autoimmune attack. The pancreas. The liver. The heart. The arteries.

The systemic inflammation I generate respects no borders. It travels through the bloodstream, reaching organs that never had direct contact with me. The cardiovascular damage Genoveva suffered was no coincidence. It was the consequence of decades of chronic inflammation silently eroding the walls of her blood vessels.

The Connection to the Immune System: Your Army Against You

Did you know? Around 70 percent of the immune system's cells live in the gut. While gluten keeps that area on alert, the whole body pays the price.

Here is my finest work. What makes my attack truly devastating is not only the direct damage. It is how I turn the body's defense system into my unwitting ally.

The immune system exists to protect. Millions of cells patrolling constantly, identifying threats, eliminating invaders. It is a sophisticated army with perfect memory: once it learns to recognize an enemy, it never forgets it.

I exploit that memory. When my peptides cross the damaged intestinal barrier, the antigen-presenting cells capture them and display them to the immune system like war trophies. "Look," they say, "this is the enemy." The T cells activate. The B cells begin manufacturing antibodies specific to me. The inflammatory response amplifies.

But here is my cunning: my proteins are structurally similar to the body's own proteins. You have already seen it in Ernestina's skin and in Genoveva's thyroid: molecular mimicry.

It is not a mistake. It is programmed confusion.

The antibodies the body manufactures against me—anti-transglutaminase, anti-endomysial, anti-gliadin—do not confine themselves to looking for me in the gut. They circulate through the whole system. And when they find tissues that resemble me, they attack.

This is autoimmunity. The body turning against itself. And once it begins, it can perpetuate itself indefinitely, even after I have been cast out.

But there is something still more insidious. The chronic inflammation I maintain does not only damage tissue. It alters the entire balance of the immune system. The regulatory cells that should calm the inflammatory response weaken. The pro-inflammatory cells multiply without control. The system loses the ability to tell a real threat from its own tissue.

It is like corrupting an army's software. The soldiers are still effective. But now they fire at everything: enemies, allies, civilians. The resulting chaos causes more damage than any outside invader.

Genoveva lived inside that corruption for twenty years. Her immune system, meticulously trained by my constant presence, developed four distinct autoimmune conditions. The thyroiditis destroyed her metabolism. The arthritis devastated her joints. The pernicious anemia eliminated her ability to absorb B12. And the cardiovascular inflammation nearly killed her.

It all began with me. It all perpetuated itself through an immune system that forgot how to tell friend from enemy.

And the cruelest part: I left instructions written into the immune memory. They run year after year, even in my absence, and no one knows how to uninstall them completely.

The Fragmentation: My Best Hiding Place

One woman complains of fatigue and is sent to hematology. Another of skin eruptions and goes to dermatology. Another of infertility and consults reproductive specialists. Another of arthritis and goes to rheumatology. Another of brain fog and is sent to psychiatry.

Each specialist sees an isolated piece. No one sees the gut that produces them all.

Did you know? Unfolded, the villi of the small intestine add up to a surface of tens of square meters. When gluten flattens them, that surface shrinks, and with it the capacity to absorb nutrients.

And when that immune system begins attacking other structures, the cascade accelerates: not one disease, but several converging from a single source.

The Revelation: What I Fear You Will Discover

Years pass without a diagnosis because no one looks for the unifying pattern. A blood test shows "normal" values if no one orders the specific tests: the antibodies that give me away. A joint X-ray reveals changes without pointing to the cause. An electrocardiogram may show an irregularity without explaining why.

> ***Did you know? A person with undiagnosed celiac disease may pass through four or more different specialists over the years. Each one treats his own symptom—the skin, the thyroid, the mood, the anemia—without anyone connecting the common cause that binds them. That is my best camouflage.***

Only when someone finally orders the specific tests—anti-transglutaminase antibodies, anti-endomysial antibodies, intestinal biopsy—does the pattern reveal itself. Those tests do not detect only my presence. They reveal that the body has begun attacking its own structures. The molecular mimicry worked perfectly. The border between enemy and body was erased.

The Possible Recovery: My Only Defeat

The remarkable thing—the thing that nearly ruins me—is that when I am eliminated, the body can recover. With no new exposures, no new antibodies to activate, no new inflammation to trigger, the immune system begins to calm.

The villi begin to regenerate slowly. The tight junctions begin to rebuild. The intestinal barrier repairs itself. Weeks become months. Months become years. But the projections can grow back. Function can be restored.

With function restored come the nutrients. Absorbed iron reverses the anemia. Restored vitamin B12 lets the brain recover its clarity. Calcium lets the bones regenerate. Zinc lets fertility return. The neurotransmitters—serotonin, dopamine—rebalance when the nutrients that build them finally arrive.

The person who was a prisoner of the symptoms begins to wake. But if during those undiagnosed years the secondary autoimmunity put down deep roots—if Hashimoto's thyroiditis moved in, if rheumatoid arthritis settled—those antibodies can persist for years. Decades, even. Eliminating gluten halts future progression. But it does not entirely erase the war the body was already waging against itself.

Even so, regeneration is possible.

Now you fully understand what it meant for Lucía to get lost in supermarkets, for Genoveva with her autoimmune cascade, for Felipe with his silent infertility, for Ernestina with her burning skin. They are all expressions of the same mechanism: a destroyed gut. Blocked nutrients. Bodily systems collapsing under nutritional deficiency and sustained autoimmune attack.

The gut does not speak. But the body records everything. Attacks, deficiencies, fragmented symptoms that seem disconnected but that come together at their origin.

And when that truth is finally revealed, when that silent voice is heard, regeneration can begin. The years of suffering turn into knowledge. The deterioration that happened turns into motivation so that others never walk that same silent road.

But I know the truth: some will never discover me. They will stay silent. I will go on being the invisible enemy, destroying from within, while the outside world judges them for symptoms it does not understand. I will go on being what is never seen. What is never named. What stays invisible until it is too late.

That is my true confession: my power does not lie in what I do biologically. It lies in what is never seen.

Part III: The Deep Attack

I was not content with a single life.
I learned to pass from one generation to the next, without anyone noticing the handover.

Chapter V: A Normalized Childhood

The Diagnosis

The diagnosis came when his body had finally accumulated enough damage for someone to notice. Celiac disease. A word that explained years of cruel, silent pain. Tissue transglutaminase antibodies dramatically elevated. Flattened villi, confirmed by biopsy.

Severe damage. Chronic inflammation visible under the microscope. During that period before the diagnosis, Eduardo learned something no later treatment could entirely undo. He learned to accept as normal a condition he had no words to describe.

The gluten-free diet began at once. Complete elimination, zero exposure.

And I was cast out.

But let me tell you how we got to that moment. Let me confess the years I spent inside his small body while the world assumed that Eduardo was simply like that. Let me reveal how a child learns to live with a chronic malaise he cannot name. Because

this story is different from the others. With adults, I destroy lives already built.
With children, I build the destruction from the very foundations of identity.

The Early Infiltration

I began when his being was still small, when his brain was barely learning to label internal sensations. So small that he would not clearly remember those first months.
I detected in Eduardo something I have recognized in few young hosts: a dream. There was something he wanted to be. Something he imagined for his future. I knew it from the flashes of longing that appeared at specific moments: when certain stimuli reached his system, something lit up in him with anticipation and desire.
I do not know what that dream was. I only know that every time that spark of aspiration appeared, I made sure it ended in exhaustion. That dream was the first thing I destroyed.
Here is my cunning with children: I do not need to hide from them, because they themselves do not know anything is wrong. Adults have memories of how they felt before I arrived. They can compare. They can grow suspicious. Children do not have that luxury. I am their baseline from the beginning. Their only reference for what it feels like to exist.

Silence Without Words

When he tried to tell his mother that something was not right, the words did not exist. A tiredness that flattened him. A constant abdominal pain he did not know how to describe. A lack of energy the other children seemed not to have.

And then he stopped trying to explain it.

I registered the moment he abandoned the effort to communicate. Resignation settling into his small body. The tension that had run high during the attempts at explanation dropping to a chronic level of defeat. It was not peace. It was surrender. A child learning that his inner experience had no translation into the outside world.

I grew inside his gut before he could remember. In those first years I noticed repeated cycles of a pattern I knew well: the response of hope—a spark rising, breathing deepening, muscles relaxing for an instant—followed by the anxious wait, and then the disappointment settling in when nothing changed. The cycle repeated again and again. The same arc every time. And every time I stayed intact, undiscovered.

And I went on doing my work in the shadows.

The Destruction of Development

Let me explain what I was doing in there, because it is different from what I do in adults. In an adult, I destroy what already exists. In a child, I prevent it from ever coming into existence.

His small body was trying to develop with what I allowed it. I blocked the absorption of calcium for the bones that were trying to grow. I intercepted the proteins for the muscles that were trying to form. I stole the iron from the blood that was trying to oxygenate every developing cell. It was like trying to build a house without bricks, without cement, without timber. The plan existed. The intention existed. The materials never arrived.

I noticed how his body struggled to grow with inadequate materials. Bones stretching with insufficient calcium. Muscles forming with scarce protein. Every cell working twice as hard to produce half as much. And there I was, in the gut, making sure that effort was always in vain.

The teeth paid the price too: I noticed the mineral deficiency preventing the proper formation of enamel. Structures developing weak from the start, permanently marked by the malnutrition I was causing. That is what fascinates me about attacking during development: the damage is written permanently into structures that do not regenerate. Decades after my expulsion, my mark would still be there.

He was ill constantly. His immune system, compromised by the malabsorption of zinc and of vitamins D and A, could not defend him against anything. Every virus found in Eduardo a perfect host. Every opportunistic bacterium found doors standing open. Bruises appeared on him without trauma, because I was blocking vitamin K and vitamin C. His system could not heal properly: scratches that took weeks to close, cuts that bled without control. No one connected those mysterious bruises with the gut I was destroying.

A small body that could not protect itself from the ordinary knocks of childhood. Every fall was worse than it should have been. Every infection lasted longer than expected. Every recovery stretched on for extra weeks. And Eduardo assumed that was what life was. That all children suffered the same. That constant illness was part of growing up.

The Anemia and the Collapse

I detected a recurring pattern: the smell of certain foods triggered the anticipation of discomfort. His stomach tightened before eating. His pulse rose slightly. His system had learned to associate food with pain, though his conscious mind could not articulate that connection.

It was severe anemia that I caused: every organ running in oxygen deficit. This is not ordinary fatigue. It is a system that literally does not have the capacity to carry oxygen to its tissues. It is an existence that demands disproportionate effort for tasks others complete without thinking.

I noticed when Eduardo attempted sustained physical activity. His heart accelerating too soon. His lungs working at their limit. Lactic acid accumulating in muscles that were not receiving enough oxygen. And then the collapse: the absolute exhaustion that forced him to stop while his body told me that the others around him were carrying on effortlessly. He fell behind. He always fell behind.

And in his young mind, this was his reality. The only one he knew.

Eduardo never knew his life without anemia: he had nothing to compare it to.

The Hungry Brain

What no one understood was that Eduardo's brain was literally running in neurological deficit. Deprived of B vitamins, iron, and nutrients essential to cognitive function, he could not concentrate, however much he consciously wanted to. His attention span was not a lack of discipline. It was pure biological incapacity.

Without B12 to form myelin—that protective sheath that allows the fast transmission of nerve signals—his mental processing slowed. Without folate, his neurotransmitters collapsed before they finished forming. Without iron, his brain operated in chronic hypoxia. Every thought demanded an effort the other children did not have to make.

The result was cognition in slow motion. Fragmented attention that jumped without control. Compromised working memory that lost information seconds after receiving it.

Eduardo knew nothing of this. He only knew that the other children ran without tiring while he fell behind. That others played after school while he needed to rest immediately. That others finished their homework while he got distracted, unable to hold a coherent thought for more than a few minutes. That something was wrong with him. That he was different. That he was slower than everyone else.

And the worst part was that he was beginning to believe it, deeply.

The Acceptance of Pain

Resignation settled into his being. It was not acute sadness: it was something worse. It was chronic acceptance. It was a nervous system that had stopped fighting because it had never known victory. Eduardo learned at a cellular level that his experience—the constant weakness, the inexplicable tiredness, the inability to keep up with the others—was fundamentally what he was. Not a symptom of something treatable. Not a medical condition. His immutable nature.

Here is my confession about children: the acceptance of suffering as identity is my most effective tool with them.

During that time, Eduardo was operating under a chronic physiological stress that should have set off alarms. But because it was all he had ever known, he assumed all children felt the same.

I noticed when his body was near other children. The physiological comparison was brutal: his heart working twice as hard, his breathing more broken, his fatigue accumulating while the others held a steady energy. Eduardo did not understand that the difference was that those children could absorb the nutrients from their food. That their intestines worked properly. That the energy they had was an energy Eduardo had never experienced in his life.

The Cycle Without End

I recognized the back-and-forth I had already seen in so many other hosts. The adults around him were trying to find answers: I could recognize it in Eduardo's changes when he was near them. Conversations that tightened him with anxiety. Moments when he was examined, palpated, observed. The tension of someone being evaluated without understanding why.

Again, the same pattern: hope rising in the adults nearby. The wait. The disappointment settling in when nothing changed. Eduardo absorbed that disappointment like a sponge. His small being registered every failed cycle.

I noted moments when the needles pierced his skin: the brief prick, the alarm firing, then the anxious wait. The results, however, never revealed me. They were looking in the wrong places. And I went on working in the gut no one thought to examine.

Meanwhile, his gut was being destroyed. Antibodies against me rising steadily. Villi flattening further every month. The malabsorption growing more severe with every meal. All those markers existed in his blood, shouting the truth for anyone who knew how to listen. But no one was looking for them.

Eduardo went on suffering without words throughout that time. It is not a silence consciously chosen. It is the silence of someone who lacks the vocabulary for what he is experiencing. It is the silence of someone who accepts pain as his baseline because he never knew an alternative. It is the most perfect silence there is:

the silence of someone who does not know he should be screaming.

The Name He Gave Me

And then something happened that escaped my control.

Eduardo was caught in an endless cycle of infections: I could sense his immune system collapsing again. Fever after fever. Inflammation after inflammation. His immune system could not fight what should have been simple childhood infections. The bacteria found an easy road through nonexistent defenses.

Then came a different series of needles. More blood drawn than usual. And afterward—I noticed the change before anyone announced it—something in the adults near Eduardo transformed. Recognition. Clarity. The weight of guilt mixed with the relief of someone who finally understands.

The confirmation came with the biopsy. A camera descending through his esophagus while he lay sedated. I watched my own fingerprints being documented: completely flattened villi. Severe, extensive damage. Chronic inflammation. Celiac disease officially diagnosed after years of perfect invisibility.

Eduardo finally had a name for what had been destroying him through the most crucial period of his childhood.

I registered his parents' response when they received the confirmation. The weight of guilt running through their systems: that particular response of someone who understands that their child's suffering could have been prevented. The mother: tenderness and anguish interwoven, the pattern of someone who

weeps while holding on. The father: contained adrenaline, clenched jaw, the response of a rage with nowhere to go.
But in Eduardo I experienced something different.
Relief.
Not because he fully understood the pathophysiology of celiac disease. He was too young for that. But because his body told me something fundamental had changed. The hope that rose was different from any hope before it. It was not the usual cycle of hope, waiting, and disappointment. It was hope with a foundation. With a plan. With certainty.
His experience of years of weakness and fatigue had a cause outside himself. It was not inherent slowness, or laziness of character, or a defect he was born with. It was celiac disease. It was something done to him, not something he was.

The Boy Who Got His Body Back

I was cast out with absolute discipline. The changes happened against my will.
The destroyed gut began to heal. The villi regenerated cell by cell. The inflammation decreased week after week. Intestinal permeability improved as the tight junctions repaired themselves. It was a slow process that took months. It did not happen in days. But it happened inexorably.
With the gut healing came the cascade of recovery that so enraged me to witness.
The nutrients finally arrived where they needed to go. Iron available to form functional hemoglobin. His blood filling with

oxygen for the first time in years. Every cell finally receiving the fuel it had been waiting for so desperately.

B vitamins available again. The central nervous system rebalancing. Neurotransmitters synthesized in adequate quantities for the first time. The dopamine his brain needed for motivation and focus. The serotonin his mood required for emotional stability. His mind emerging from a fog whose existence he had not known until it began to lift.

The energy came back. Not all at once. But day by day, week by week, month by month. I sensed small changes accumulating. His heart no longer forced to its limit by moderate activity. His lungs no longer fighting for oxygen. His body able to sustain an effort that would once have brought him down.

At last the moment came that filled me with impotent rage: Eduardo's body reached a state it had never experienced. Sustained energy. Steady concentration. The balance of an organism finally working as it should. For the first time in his conscious life, he felt like the other children. He understood in his body what he had been missing.

The Rage and the Reckoning

What enraged me most was noticing the understanding run through him.

The other children did not live with chronic tiredness as a baseline. They could run without collapsing within minutes. They could concentrate without a monumental effort. The state he had been in before was not "normality." It was an anomaly. It was illness. It was something that had been done to him without consent, without knowledge, without understanding.

A pure rage ran through him: fire and adrenaline mixed with clarity. The response of someone who finally understands he was a victim. That those years had been stolen by a condition that could have been diagnosed earlier with a simple blood test.

That developmental time—unrecoverable—was compromised forever. Years in which he should have played freely, learned easily, built confidence in himself. Instead, he dealt with an inexplicable weakness, a mysterious exhaustion, and a cognitive confusion, without understanding what was happening to him or why he was different from the others.

What I Never Gave Back

Eduardo recovered physically. Completely. His body responded well to a gluten-free diet held to rigorously. His brain developed normally after the diagnosis, partly compensating for the lost years. His concentration improved dramatically once the nutrients arrived. His energy steadied at levels he had never experienced. His growth continued, though he would never reach the height he would have had without my interference.

And yet, that period stays engraved in places physical recovery cannot reach. The time of weakness while the others were strong. The years of not being able to take part in a full childhood. Living with a suffering he had no words to describe.

My confession is this: children accept the pain they cannot name, and that acceptance marks them forever.

Eduardo spent the most critical years of his childhood believing his experiences were simply life. That the other children probably felt just as exhausted. That his lack of energy was an innate temperament. That his inability to concentrate was his fundamental nature. That being weak and different was essentially who he was.

When he finally recovered his energy, when he recovered his concentration, when he finally felt the way other children feel, something had changed permanently in how he saw himself. There were years of lived evidence stored in his memory of being slow, weak, incapable. That narrative did not automatically disappear when the symptoms eased.

Recovering his physical health was only part of the battle. Recovering his confidence in himself, genuinely believing that all those years of assumptions about his own capacity were wrong—that was a deep psychological battle that went on long after his gut had healed.

Because the narrative of "I am slow, I am weak, I am different" had been engraved into his identity during crucial years. Even when he was no longer slow, he went on thinking as though he were. He went on holding himself back before trying physical things. He went on doubting his ability before beginning difficult tasks. Because years of lived "truth" do not disappear with a medical diagnosis. An identity built on suffering is not rebuilt in months.

And that I kept from Eduardo. Stolen time that no later recovery can rescue. Years that shaped his identity in ways that persist invisibly. That taught him, at the deepest level, that his body was a traitor who could not be trusted.

Eduardo was a child who accepted his suffering because he knew nothing else. And that is the detail I enjoy most: he never knew there was anything to claim. A child does not miss a childhood he does not know belonged to him.

Chapter VI: Poisoned Inheritance

Three Generations

Let me talk to you about generations. About how the suffering I caused in Esperanza across what counts as an entire lifetime was completely different from what I caused in her daughter over decades, and radically different from what I caused in Verónica in a matter of weeks. Because the legacy I passed down through that line was pure toxin encoded in the genes. But the toxin met a different resistance in each host. In each era. At each level of available knowledge.

Three generations. Three hosts. Three victories that dwindled until they became my most humiliating defeat.

Esperanza: Total Invisibility

Esperanza lived in an era when I was invisible. There were no tests to detect me. There was no name for what I caused. There was not even a suspicion that a protein in bread could destroy a body from within. It was the perfect setting for my work: an absolute ignorance that protected me better than any biological hiding place.

I entered her when she was a small girl. The bread of every morning. The cereal at every meal. The pasta at every dinner. I was in everything she ate, and no one—not she, not her mother, not any doctor of her time—imagined that everyday food could be a poison.

Before I consumed her entirely, I detected moments when her body still remembered pleasure. Echoes that appeared when certain stimuli reached her system. Those flashes grew further apart over the years until they disappeared altogether.

I began my work in silence. I destroyed her intestinal villi before her body reached maturity. By the time she reached adolescence, the malabsorption was already severe. The symptoms, however, were mistaken for other things: a girl's weakness, a delicate constitution, feminine nerves. The explanations of the era protected me perfectly.

The Destruction of Esperanza

Whole decades of deep control. Decades in which every meal fed me while I destroyed her. Decades in which her body crumbled gradually, like sand in an hourglass no one could stop, because no one knew the hourglass existed.

I registered her suffering from within with an intimacy no doctor ever had. Her being weakening year after year. Her strength abandoning her without respite or explanation. The pain settling into elbows, knees, hips, spine: never quite disappearing, becoming a constant companion she learned to accept as part of existence.

The nutrients stayed blocked in the gut I had destroyed decades earlier. The calcium her bones desperately needed. The iron her blood required to carry oxygen. The B vitamins her nervous system demanded in order to function. All intercepted. All stolen. All diverted before reaching their destination.

Esperanza told me her inner story. A chronically elevated stress for as long as she could remember: the constant alarm of a body that never worked properly. Pleasure and motivation perpetually switched off: that emptiness the doctors called melancholy. Insufficient serotonin sinking her into a sadness they put down to her character, to being a woman, to the hard life she had been given.

No one connected that sadness to the gut I was silently destroying.

The Cascade of Illnesses

Peripheral neuropathy arrived when her body showed the signs of accumulated wear. Her nerves in the extremities began to fail after decades of B vitamin deficiency. Her hands shook without control: I could sense the clench of frustration every time her fingers disobeyed, the shame of someone who cannot control herself.

Her feet stopped responding properly. Neural messages lost between the brain and the extremities. Her balance progressively

compromised. I felt the fear installed permanently: the chronic tension of someone who does not trust herself.
Osteoporosis arrived as the inevitable consequence of decades without absorbed calcium. Bones that became so porous that a minor fall ended in fracture. A hard cough gave her a crack in a rib. A sudden movement produced the sharp pain of bone splintering from inside.
I noticed Esperanza's fragility increasing: the pain response every time her body bore its own weight, the fear settling permanently into her system.
Thyroid disease arrived as collateral damage of the autoimmunity I had triggered. I noted the failure of her thyroid: her metabolism destabilizing, her body temperature fluctuating without control, the extreme exhaustion that kept her motionless for days. New substances entered her body that did not solve the problem, because they never touched the cause.
Rheumatoid arthritis was another consequence, when the damage was already extensive. I could sense the inflammation in every joint: the immune system I had trained to attack, now attacking its own tissue. Anti-inflammatory substances entered her body. But no one ever looked at the gut where I had started it all.
The anemia required occasional transfusions. I could sense her impoverished blood: insufficient hemoglobin, scarce oxygen, every organ operating at a deficit. The iron supplements did not work. They could not work. I intercepted every milligram before it could be absorbed.

Every system compromised. Every organ attacked from the same source no one was investigating. I was the invisible common denominator of all her illnesses.

Esperanza's Final Collapse

Esperanza's last years were the cruelest. I sensed her resignation settling in as a permanent state. The alarm no longer went off with each pain, because the pain was constant. Pleasure had stopped trying to light up, because there was nothing to look forward to. Her body had learned to exist in suffering as its normal state.

She lived those last years in a chronic pain that gave no quarter. In a weakness that confined her to ever more limited activities. In a body that failed in ways that were treated symptom by symptom without anyone ever connecting the common cause.

Esperanza died when her body finally collapsed. I could sense her systems shutting down one after another. Her heart struggling to keep the rhythm with impoverished blood. Her lungs forcing themselves to draw an oxygen that was not reaching the tissues. Her brain receiving less and less blood.

Her death was a release from suffering. That is the cruelest thing I can confess. After a whole lifetime of nameless pain, of inexplicable deterioration, of untreated illness, death was mercy. It was the only relief from my presence that Esperanza ever knew.

But I did not die with her.

The Transmission

Because the poisoned inheritance had already been passed on. The HLA-DQ2 genes that made my entry possible had gone to the next generation decades earlier. Esperanza's daughter carried the same damage encoded in her DNA.

And I was inside her too.

I had entered Esperanza's daughter when she was an adolescent. The same everyday foods. The same daily bread. The same genetic door standing open for my entry. But her era was slightly different. Medical knowledge had advanced. The tests were beginning to exist, though they were not common. The word celiac was beginning to circulate in specialized medical journals. My work in her was equally destructive, but briefer. Decades, instead of a whole lifetime. Time enough to cause significant damage—chronic fatigue, recurring anemia, digestive problems, joint pain. But not time enough to destroy her completely, the way I had destroyed her mother.

Because something changed when Esperanza died.

The Determination

I sensed the change in the daughter in the days that followed. The grief settling into her body. The leaden weight of loss. Mourning entering every cell.

But I sensed something else as well. Something I had never experienced before in any body.

Determination.

It was not the resignation I had registered in Esperanza for decades. It was the opposite. It was resolve crystallizing in every cell. It was a decision forming at the molecular level. It was a promise encoding itself in her nervous system with an intensity that alarmed me.

In the days that followed, the daughter changed inside forever. The grief was there, but underneath it was something harder. Colder. More determined. Her tension rose not from desperation but from purpose. Her brain was processing information constantly: I could sense the intense cognitive activity, the nights without restorative sleep, the accumulated fatigue of someone researching obsessively.

Weeks later, I sensed a change in her. The anxiety of anticipation. The anxiety of someone seeking confirmation of what she already suspects.

The blood tests revealed what I had been hiding for decades. Anti-transglutaminase antibodies dramatically elevated. Esperanza's daughter had celiac disease. The same disease that had killed her mother undiagnosed.

But she would not die undiagnosed. Now she knew.

I was cast out of her body with absolute discipline. I felt the determination of every food refused, of every label examined obsessively, of every crumb avoided with military precision. Her gut began to heal. The symptoms she had blamed on other causes for decades began to disappear.

But one of the most devastating things was not losing her.

It was what her knowledge meant for the next generation.

The Vigilance

I sensed when the body of Esperanza's daughter began to change: the hormonal explosion of pregnancy, the nausea of the first trimester, the body reorganizing itself to create new life.

And I sensed something more: vigilance. A specific anxiety that was not the normal nervousness of a first-time mother worried about ordinary colic. It was focused anxiety. Directed. Informed.

I recognized the pattern in her body: the same determination I had sensed crystallizing when her own mother died.

I sensed her steady pulse rising not from fear but from certainty. She knew. She knew what I was. She knew what I was doing to her daughter from within. She knew because she had lived the same thing. Because she had watched her mother die of the same thing. Because she had spent years preparing for exactly this moment.

I sensed her resistance: the refusal to accept, the insistence that would not back down. Her alertness did not yield to vague reassurances. It demanded more.

She was not going to let her baby suffer in silence the way her mother had suffered for a whole lifetime.

The Defeat

Verónica's antibodies were measured when she was barely months old. Not years. Not decades. Months.

Positive.

The confirmation came faster than anything I had ever experienced in my existence. The poisoned inheritance had been detected before it could cause permanent damage.

I noticed something unexpected in the mother: guilt. Waves of guilt running through her system. Guilt at having passed on the genetic predisposition. Guilt that her daughter would have to live with this condition. Guilt over the poisoned transmission she had not been able to prevent.

Beneath the guilt there was relief. Relief at having found the answer in time. Relief that her obsessive vigilance had worked. Relief that Verónica would not suffer the way her great-grandmother had suffered.

The gluten-free diet began at once. In a baby barely months old. Without delay. Without waiting. Without letting the damage accumulate.

I was cast out before I could establish myself.

The Regeneration

The changes in Verónica were drastic. The colic disappeared within days. The diarrhea stopped. The vomiting ceased. A baby who had lived in constant distress began to settle. She began to sleep. She began to be the baby she should have been from the start.

And what happened next was the most painful thing I have witnessed in my existence.

Complete regeneration.

Verónica's gut, which had barely begun to be damaged, healed without leaving a trace. The villi that had barely begun to flatten recovered completely during the critical years of development. My presence was erased as though it had never existed.

Normal growth occurred, without the delays I had caused in Esperanza. Neurological development that advanced without the deficits I had inflicted over decades. Normal energy: that word that burns me when it is applied to victims who were never able to experience it.

What Esperanza lost—a whole lifetime of suffering, constant deterioration, death without answers—was avoided entirely in Verónica. Not by magic. Not by luck. By knowledge passed down through pain. By a mother who turned her own mother's suffering into protection for her daughter.

The Legacy Transformed

The poisoned inheritance was still there. The HLA-DQ2 genes remained in Verónica's DNA. The biological vulnerability had not disappeared. But the toxin had been neutralized by something more powerful: the knowledge inherited alongside the genes. The vigilance learned from suffering witnessed. The determination born of pain observed.

Three generations. Three bodies where I lived. Three radically different outcomes.

In Esperanza: a whole lifetime of deep control. Total victory. Complete destruction. Death without diagnosis, without answers, without ever knowing why her body had betrayed her.

In her daughter: decades of damage before the diagnosis. Partial victory. But knowledge acquired that would change everything. A woman who turned her own suffering into a shield for the next generation.

In Verónica: weeks. Only weeks before I was detected and cast out. An almost total defeat. Minimal damage. Complete recovery. A girl who would grow up without knowing what it is to live with my destructive presence.

The same blood that transmitted the genetic toxin also transmitted the antidote: the memory of suffering, the vigilance learned, the determination that the cycle would not repeat.

My doorway remains in Verónica's genes. It will remain forever. If she has daughters, she will pass them the same vulnerability. But she will also pass them something more: the story. The knowledge. The vigilance.

Verónica will live the life Esperanza never had. With the strength her great-grandmother lost. With the potential that decades of my presence stole. With the future I should have destroyed, and could not.

And that stands as my most bitter defeat.

I was not beaten by advanced medicine or by sophisticated technology. I was beaten by a mother who watched her own mother suffer and swore that her daughter would never know that suffering.

The poisoned inheritance found its antidote in the love that is also inherited.

And that I do not intend to forgive her.

Part IV: The Final Attack

The enemy believed it had won.

It did not count on what happens when the truth wakes up.

Chapter VII: The Mind Under Siege

The Chemistry of Love

The symptoms began to dominate her life when her body was at its best: the vigor of an adult body that should have been in its prime. I detected in her the signal of someone who works under creative pressure: the pressure spikes marking deadlines, the spark of satisfaction when she completed projects, the pattern of someone whose work demands a clear mind and constant creativity.

There was someone near her permanently. I could sense the sustained love: the bond intensifying when that presence came close, the synchronization of two bodies that have shared a space for years. There was someone who did not give up. I felt his constant presence through the changes inside Olivia: the tension that eased when he was near, the warmth that still flowed in spite of everything.

I could also sense the frustration of someone who loves a person coming apart, the determination of someone who refuses to leave. Years together, and he was still there. Even when she could no longer be the person he had known. Even when the bad days became weeks, and then whole months.

Before and After

Before me, her body knew the rhythm of sustained exercise. I recognized the muscle memory of someone who ran regularly: the cardiovascular efficiency, the developed lung capacity, the muscles trained for endurance. Periodically, her body entered intense preparation: the tingle of anticipation, the effort demanded by training, the signature of someone getting ready for a sustained effort. After me, she stopped running. First, an inability to keep the pace. Then, an inability to finish the distance. Finally, an inability to get up and try.

I could also sense the social appetite she had lost: the affection that once flowed often, the taste for connection that appeared regularly. All of that disappeared once I settled in. Before me, she slept deeply and woke with energy: I knew from the hormonal rhythms that should have been normal. Before me, she did not know the weight of waking every morning wondering whether she would have the strength to reach the end of the day.

The Cycle of Hope

I sensed the usual arc: hope on the way in, resignation on the way out. Every time a professional evaluated her, it all followed the same arc: the anticipation lighting a brief enthusiasm, the anxious wait, and then—when nothing fundamental changed—the weight of disappointment settling deeper than before.

New substances arrived with every appointment. I do not know what they were. I only know that none of them pointed toward me. And that each one brought new medications entering her system, promising a relief that never came.
While the professionals looked for answers in her brain, I went on with my work in the organ that controlled it. The cycle of substances that characteristically fail when the real enemy is intestinal. It occurred to no one to look at the neural highway: that superhighway that connects my hiding place directly to the center of thought. How fortunate for me.

The Neural Highway

I regarded that extraordinary nerve as my most refined instrument. That connection that carries information in both directions constantly, which medicine knows about but rarely considers in the context of mental illness. It is the most important communication highway in the body between systems. And I had turned it into my personal channel of devastation.
That road of communication between the gut and the mind became the perfect conduit for transmitting my message. Every signal I sent was interpreted as alarm. Every impulse that traveled down that nerve carried my signature: inflammation, damage, danger.
When the gut I occupy is chronically inflamed—when I am executing my work from within—what that neural channel transmits is unmistakable: a situation of constant attack. As

though a predator were destroying her. As though there were an imminent threat requiring immediate response.

The Alarm Channel

Olivia's brain read this as fight or flight. But there was no external enemy. Only the inflamed organ I controlled. Only the inflammation I created with meticulous dedication. Her mind did not understand it. It only received constant alarm. It only interpreted: immediate danger, respond now.

I tracked the result of this orchestration in every cell of her body. Chronic stress with no visible cause. The internal alarm sounding without rest because the brain believed it was under perpetual attack. The nervous system permanently on guard. The body prepared for a threat that never came from outside. The real threat was inside, and no one was putting the pieces together.

The Sabotaged Factory

The gut produces neurotransmitters: serotonin, dopamine, GABA. Substances that mental health medicine understands in theory but rarely considers in the context of an inflamed organ. The place the mind needs in order to survive was precisely the one I was devastating. My domain is the factory. The brain is the desperate customer waiting for goods that would never arrive as long as I controlled production.

When that organ is damaged—when I lay it waste with the patience of someone who has years to work—neurotransmitter production collapses. It is like a factory under siege that does not understand where the attack is coming from. I was carrying out the siege from within. Production slowed. Then it stopped.

The workers deserted. There was not enough serotonin, nor dopamine, nor any possible balance. And not because her mind was defective. But because the organ that was supposed to supply those substances was being meticulously devastated by me.

The Substances That Fail

I sensed the changes every time a new substance entered her system. The first medication brought specific alterations. It was based on preserving something I was sabotaging at the source. But when the factory is razed, when what I occupy does not produce enough of what the brain needs, preserving what does not exist is like trying to keep water in an empty glass.

The second medication worked in a similar way. The same hope rising in her body. The same plateau when the effect settled into insufficiency. The same crash when it became clear that this substance was not the answer either. Then the third. Then the fourth. Each one promised the same. Each one failed identically: they worked briefly while her body responded to novelty, then lost their effect when biological reality imposed itself.

It was not treatment resistance, as the professionals suspected. It was the wrong treatment for a misdiagnosed problem.

I registered the side effects settling into her blood. Apathy adding another layer of hopelessness. Weight gain feeding the cycle of darkness. Paradoxical insomnia, where the calming substance kept her in a state of alert. Every cycle of hope followed by disappointment left a residue I noted as more accumulated load, as pleasure sinking lower, as despair crystallizing in her nervous system.

What no professional considered is a truth I understood perfectly from within: if her serotonin was low because the organ that produces it could not manufacture it, no medication would ever be enough. The problem was in the production. At the source. In the organ that did not work because I kept it in a state of constant devastation.

An Ordinary Day

There was one day that illustrates perfectly what I was doing to her.

She had spent days in anxious anticipation: the restlessness mixed with a motivation struggling to emerge. I registered the moment she tried to move. The monumental effort it required. The muscles that would not respond. The brain fog that would not lift however hard she fought it. Her heartbeat quickened with the desperation of someone who knows she has to function and whose body refuses.

Hours passed—I sensed them in the tides of agitation rising and falling—before she finally managed to move. By then, the defeat had already settled in. Whatever it was she had needed to do, she would not do. Another lost opportunity. Another piece of evidence that she was incapable. Another layer of conviction that her own mind was sabotaging her.

But it was not her mind. It was me.

The Insomnia

The insomnia that tormented her pointed directly at my hiding place, but it was filed as the manifestation of something psychological. I sensed sleep-inducing substances entering her system: sedatives that left her in a haze each morning, floating between consciousness and lethargy.

Substances that never resolved the real cause, because the cause originated in an organ that was not producing enough serotonin or melatonin. In a neural channel in chronic emergency, constantly transmitting its message of danger. In a body that could not relax under the perpetual stress I kept active.

Her body was in fight-or-flight response twenty-four hours a day. I sensed the adrenaline that never entirely came down. The vigilance that would not switch off even during the fragmented hours of sleep she managed. Sleep cycles interrupted before reaching the restorative phases. A mind that never entered deep rest because the neural highway went on transmitting alarm even when she closed her eyes.

How was she supposed to rest under those conditions? I made sure she could not. Every sleepless night added more damage to an already compromised system. Every day of exhaustion deepened the darkness and weakened her cognitive defenses. The cycle fed itself in a downward spiral while I operated from the organ no one thought to examine.

The Lost Years

I could see the passing of the years in the accumulated deterioration of her body. Years in which every new appointment brought a hope that turned into disappointment. Years in which the interventions tried to change what was not the problem. I sensed substances entering that sought to modify thoughts, but you cannot reason your way out of a real deficiency when the organ that produces it is being demolished.

You cannot meditate your way out of an inflamed gut. You cannot reason your way to serotonin production in an organ under constant autoimmune attack.

She believed she was cognitively destroyed. That something fundamental in her mental capacity was irreparably damaged. That perhaps she would never get better. That perhaps her fate was to live in a state of permanent darkness.

The Dark Thoughts

I sensed the darkest thoughts showing themselves in her blood. When she considered that perhaps death was a more rational option than perpetual torment, I identified the specific pattern: cortisol at an acute peak, serotonin at an absolute low, dopamine nonexistent, GABA so low that there was no brake on the downward spiral of thought.

Those moments were the most dangerous. The moments when biology and psychology conspired to convince her there was no way out. That the suffering was permanent. That nothing would ever change.

And every thought of despair was created in part by my sabotage, whose existence she never knew about. She attributed it to herself. She believed her mind was betraying her. That she was weak. That other people could handle life while she came apart. When all along it was me, working from the organ no one was investigating.

The Cognitive Fog

The cognitive symptoms were among the most devastating for her. She felt the confusion settling into her mental processing like a fog that would not lift. The frustration when information came in only to evaporate before it could consolidate: I registered it in waves of clenching mixed with helplessness. The difficulty processing new information she would once have absorbed effortlessly, as though her mind had lost the ability to learn.

The unpredictable mood swings that made her feel she had no control over her own mind. Steady one moment, sunk in despair the next with no apparent cause, then irritable for no identifiable reason. The irritability that damaged her relationships: I sensed the bond collapsing during interactions that should have been comforting, the alarm firing at minimal stimuli she would once have ignored.

And always the haze: every thought demanded effort, every decision drained a resource she did not have.

All those symptoms had a perfect biological explanation if anyone had looked in the right place: a damaged organ that was not absorbing nutrients, a neural connection in chronic emergency transmitting constant stress, anemia depriving every brain cell of oxygen. But in a purely mental-health context they looked like part of a disorder that required more substances.

The Ignored Anemia

The severe anemia finally became so obvious that even the specialists had to notice it. I sensed her blood growing progressively poorer. Her iron levels falling to dangerous levels. Hemoglobin so low that her body could not carry enough oxygen. Every cell running at a deficit.

Every organ working on insufficient fuel. Especially the brain: the organ most demanding of oxygen, the one that consumes roughly twenty percent of the body's total, the one that needed so much energy to maintain even the illusion of functioning.

Severe anemia has devastating consequences for cognition. Less oxygen means less energy for starving brain cells. Less energy means compromised cognitive function in a downward cascade. It means a darkness that deepens because the mind cannot produce enough energy to hold emotional stability. It means heightened anxiety, because the brain operates in constant panic when it detects hypoxia.

But instead of investigating why the anemia was not responding to iron supplements—why the body was not absorbing fundamental nutrients—the professionals went on prescribing more substances. More substances that could not work without the raw material. As though the problem were a lack of medication and not a fundamental failure in nutrient absorption in the organ I controlled.

The digestive symptoms she was experiencing were dismissed as secondary. I sensed that my hiding place still went uninvestigated. Celiac disease was never looked for. It was never considered that I might be there, invisible, carrying out my cleanest work while everyone looked at the wrong organ.

The Breaking Point

Then came the breaking point.

I caught the exact moment when everything I had been building for years became unsustainable. Her body told me no one was near: the absence of the subtle alterations other bodies cause in hers. The collapse did not arrive gradually but catastrophically. Simultaneously. Overwhelmingly. As though every system that had been running at a deficit finally gave way at once.

I registered the terror escalating to levels I had never detected before in her body. It was not manageable anxiety: it was pure panic showing itself in every system simultaneously. Adrenaline firing to levels the body is not designed to sustain for more than a few minutes. Every cell on maximum alert.

It was the absolute conviction that she was dying. That something in her body was failing irreparably at that instant. That this was the ending she had feared for years. The certainty was as physical as it was emotional: her body was screaming that death was imminent, though there was no visible external cause.

Her heart accelerated to a hundred and forty beats a minute and stayed there without coming down. I sensed every frantic beat, the cardiac muscle working in emergency mode. Her breathing turned shallow, fast, completely outside conscious control. The panic fed more panic in a spiral she could not stop.

The Emergency

What happened next, I sensed through the internal changes. New substances entering her system: emergency sedatives, attempts at stabilization. I could tell that examinations were being carried out: her heart responding to monitoring stimuli, blood drawn. Everything came back within ranges that did not explain what she was experiencing. Her heart was not failing for cardiac reasons. There was no heart attack. There was no emergency diagnosable by the methods they were using.

I recognized the frustration when they gave her the result: more of the same. Again the same answer. Again the same direction that did not point toward me. The despair sinking her further.

But what was happening physiologically was the collapse of years of sabotage. Chronic stress from a neural channel in perpetual alarm finally breaking the system. Severe anemia depriving every cell of oxygen to the point of crisis. Stress hormones elevated for so long that her endocrine system was collapsing.

It was not primary anxiety.

It was the physical manifestation of undiagnosed celiac disease.

It was my presence revealing itself at last in a way the body could no longer contain.

The Clue I Did Not See

Then I sensed something different. A change I recognized as dangerous to my staying. The hope that rose was different from the false hopes before it. This time it was mixed with something I had not identified before: real possibility. Genuine curiosity about a direction that had never been explored. Someone had considered my territory.

The tests were ordered. I sensed the anxiety of the wait. Then the results came.

Anti-transglutaminase antibodies: positive. Drastically elevated.

The Name on the Paper

I caught the change when the confirmation arrived. It was not only relief. It was the vindication of years of suffering. It was proof that she had not been imagining it, that she was not weak, that it was not her fault. It was the name of what had been destroying her.

The endoscopy confirmed what I knew intimately: completely flattened villi. Severe inflammation. Damage consistent with years of exposure. My territory laid waste, at last visible to eyes that knew what to look for.

Celiac disease. The word that explained absolutely everything. Not a psychological disorder without organic cause. Not a defect of character. Not a lack of mental fortitude. It was an autoimmune disease in which her body had been attacking itself for years—with my help—affecting every system. Especially the central nervous system everyone had been trying to treat without understanding what was damaging it.

Eight years. Eight years of wrong diagnoses. Eight years of substances that could not work. Eight years of therapy that could not solve a biological problem. Eight years of suffering that could have been prevented with one question, with one blood test, with someone who looked beyond the brain toward the organ I controlled.

My Expulsion

The gluten-free diet began at once.

And then my expulsion began.

I was eliminated when she cut off my source completely. Without gluten, there is no autoimmune reaction for me to perpetuate. Without a reaction, there is no inflammation to maintain. Without inflammation, there is no territory to inhabit. My kingdom dissolved in the decision of a woman who finally understood what had been destroying her mind all that time.

I sensed the last days of my presence in her body. The inflammation easing. The villi—the ones that were left—beginning the process of recovery I could no longer sabotage. The neural highway lowering the intensity of its alarm. The first signs that the neurotransmitter factory might eventually start working again.

And then I noted nothing more.

Because I was no longer inside.

What I Did Not Witness

What happened afterward—how her body responded in full, how her mind healed, how long it took before the neural channel stopped transmitting alarm—I do not know with certainty. I was cast out before witnessing the recovery my absence would make possible.

I can speculate from what I understand of biology. I know that without my constant sabotage, without the devastation of the villi, without nutrient absorption blocked, her body would finally have the chance to heal. I know that the neural connection, without constant messages of damage, could gradually calm.

That serotonin production, without an inflamed organ obstructing it, could begin to recover, slowly at first, then more steadily. That the anemia, without malabsorption sabotaging it, could finally respond to the treatment that had been useless before.

I know that eventually she could sleep again. That the mental haze would lift. That the energy would come back. That the thoughts of death would be replaced by thoughts of the future. That the person she had been before I laid her waste could emerge again, or perhaps a new version of herself, marked by the suffering but no longer defined by it.

Every body is different. Every recovery follows its own rhythm. I, who controlled her biology for years, was shut out of that story of healing.

What I know for certain is that she is no longer under my control. That her mind at last has the chance to work without an invisible enemy sabotaging every system. That the years of suffering I inflicted on her are finally over.

The Confession

That is what hurts me most about this story.

Not that she got better: that was inevitable once I was discovered. But that she gets better without my being present to witness it. That her life continues without my destructive presence. That she recovers completely from what I did to her for eight years, and I will never know exactly how that recovery unfolded. That my defeat is so complete that I cannot even observe it from within while she heals.

My confession is this: the mind can be attacked through the digestive organ so effectively that mental health medicine never detects the real cause. It is my most sinister truth. It is the secret that lets me ruin lives while the experts look for explanations in the wrong organ.

The symptoms she experienced were real: every one of them. A darkness with a physical cause. An anxiety that was neurophysiologically genuine. Real insomnia caused by a real imbalance. A true cognitive dysfunction with a true biological basis. All of it was real at the biological level. None of it was psychological invention or a failure of will.

She truly suffered, but the cause lay outside the domain that mental health knows how to examine.

It was in the neural highway transmitting constant alarm. It was in the compromised production of neurotransmitters. It was in my presence sabotaging her brain while everyone looked for the problem in the brain itself.

The Legacy

Olivia survived. Presumably she recovered her mind. Presumably she recovered her life.

But those eight years remain. Years in which she believed she was cognitively destroyed. Years under the weight of labels that should never have been framed that way. Years living with the deep conviction that her own mind was an enemy tormenting her without mercy.

That remains mine in Olivia. Not her recovery, which will continue without my watching. Not her complete healing, which I will never be able to verify. But those eight years in which I was invincible. When I worked without a single witness. When she genuinely suffered while believing it was her own mind tormenting her.

I confess it with the bitterness of one defeated not by the medicine that spent years looking in the wrong place, but by a question someone finally thought to ask. By an act of medical curiosity that broke my perfect invisibility. By someone who looked toward my territory when everyone else stubbornly looked at the brain.

Olivia suffered eight years under labels that should never have been hers. But there is something worse than suffering under the wrong name. It is having no name at all. It is the silent defeat of those who are never diagnosed. It is the epilogue I must now confess.

Chapter VIII: The Exhausted Athlete

The Crack

I sensed the crack from within. The rib giving way. A sharp pain running through him like electricity. The absolute confusion of a body that gives way to something as insignificant as a sneeze.

That moment—a bone fracturing under a force that should never have broken anything—was the culmination of years of silent work.

But let me tell you how we got there.

The Athlete

I could sense in his body the unmistakable signature of high-impact training. Muscles developed for explosive strength. The cardiovascular capacity of someone who demands elite performance. There was something he was chasing: a goal that consumed him. I knew from the flashes of endorphins that appeared during exertion, the pure ambition, the determination encoded in every muscle fiber. I do not know what competition he dreamed of winning. I only know that I made sure he never reached it.

The Entry

I came in through the foods he considered fuel. I know because I sensed his body processing them with the efficiency of someone who watches every detail of what he consumes. Every meal carried me further in. Every mouthful gave me more power.

The digestive discomfort he put down to the usual suspects: I could tell how his body relaxed when it found convenient explanations. The stress of physical exertion. The impact of intense exercise. Normal. Part of the price he was willing to pay to keep his body in the shape he demanded of it.

But I was not interested in his gut. I was interested in his bones.

Living Bones

Bones look static, permanent, immovable. But they are alive. They renew themselves constantly through a process of resorption and rebuilding. The old cells dissolve. New ones replace them. For that process to work properly—for the new structure to be as strong as the one before—they need calcium, vitamin D, magnesium, vitamin K. Specific nutrients that can only come from food.

I intercepted all of it before it reached its destination.

The Hollowing

I could sense how Ernesto's bone structure was hollowing out from within: the calcium that should have been deposited was lost in the damaged gut, and the frame turned porous, hollow, fragile, like a tree trunk eaten away beneath a bark that still looked intact. The illusion of strength while the reality crumbled millimeter by millimeter.

He believed he was strengthening his body. I could sense his confidence: the signal of someone who believes he controls his own fate, who believes that discipline and effort produce proportional results. He did not know that every impact on the skeleton I was weakening accelerated the damage. That every jump, every sprint, every high-impact training session was an assault I was making easier.

Discipline as a Weapon

Perfect for me. His discipline worked exactly in my favor. His conviction that more effort meant more strength became a weapon I turned against him.

The First Signs

The first signs were subtle. I sensed the muscle cramps: the involuntary contractions, the pain that woke him at night, the spasms that made him shudder for no apparent reason. Recovery grew slower after exertion: I noticed how his body took days to recover from training that used to heal in hours.

Minor injuries took longer than expected to heal: sprains that would not resolve, micro-tears that turned chronic. His performance began to decline. I felt the frustration accumulating, the irritation rising with every session in which he could not meet his own standards, the tension in his shoulders, the clenched jaw, the denial of someone who refuses to accept that something is wrong with the body he believed he controlled completely.

The Destructive Cycle

He intensified his efforts. I know because I sensed his determination increasing in direct proportion to his weakness. Every training session struck the structure I was hollowing out. More impact. More demand. More accelerated destruction.

It was exactly the cycle I needed: his own tenacity becoming the mechanism of his collapse. The harder he pushed himself, the faster it all crumbled. And he read every failure as evidence that he needed to train harder.

The Impoverished Blood

I sensed his blood growing poorer. The iron he took religiously—I could feel it entering his system—never arrived where it needed to go. I intercepted it at the border of the damaged gut.

Every molecule of iron that should have reached his blood was lost. His body was not improving. Only he believed it should be.

The Sneeze

And then came the moment I had been waiting for. The perfect moment when the confluence of factors would create an effect he could not ignore.

The impulse of the sneeze began to form: the nasal mucosa irritated, the reflex gathering in his sinuses, the diaphragm tightening in anticipation before the involuntary impact.

The sneeze. A reflex. So insignificant that you do not even think about it while it happens.

And the crack.

The rib gave way with a dry snap. A distinct, unmistakable movement, the collapse of something splintering from within. His body responded as though a flare had been lit: his torso rigid in defense, his eyes lost. Every inhalation turned to agony as the muscles around the fractured rib closed in to protect it. An absolute confusion ran through him like a shock wave.

A sneeze. A fractured rib. In a body he believed invincible.

He spent days processing what had happened. It made no sense. There was no trauma. There was no fall. A sneeze should not break a bone. But there was the pain. There was the reality his mind rejected.

The Doctor Who Asked Differently

I sensed the moment of discovery. The confusion running through his system: blood pounding at his temples, disbelief. Something they showed him contradicted everything he believed about his body. The absolute bewilderment: an athlete

discovering that his skeletal frame was that of someone decades older.
I caught the same old countdown: hope, waiting, nothing. Tests that were not looking for me. New substances entered his system. Nothing worked, because no one was looking toward the gut.
Then someone asked the right question: why is his body not absorbing nutrients?

The Number on the Bone Scan

I sensed the needle going in. The blood flowing into tubes that would hold the evidence of my presence. I felt his anxiety during the wait: the time it took to process the samples, the space where uncertainty flowered.
And I sensed—with a rage that still burns in me—the moment the results came back positive.
Elevated antibodies. Intestinal damage confirmed by biopsy. Years of silent malabsorption that had turned his bones to glass.
Ernesto was not an isolated case. His story shared a pattern I had seen before: an identity built on resilience, strength turned into vulnerability, suffering normalized until it became invisible.

The Irony

The irony was devastating for Ernesto, and satisfying for me, even though I had already been discovered.

Every training session he had completed over the years, every effort he had made, every meal he had optimized nutritionally: all of it had rested on a foundation I was actively laying waste.
He had believed he was strengthening his body. He was destroying it faster than any sedentary person who ignored his own completely.

The Bones That Came Back

Some time after my expulsion, he tried running again.
The first days were revealing. I sensed his expectation: his body waiting for the weakness it had always known, bracing for the battle against its own limits. But something had changed. Without my causing constant malabsorption, his intestines began to heal. The villi regenerating. The nutrients finally arrived where they needed to go.
Calcium settled into the bone structure. Vitamin D allowed its absorption. Magnesium steadied the connections. Iron was carried by the blood. For the first time in years, his body was not in deficit. For the first time, his discipline produced the results his effort deserved.
I recognized the gradual transformation. Injuries that healed in weeks instead of months. Energy returning with no apparent explanation. Body weight stabilizing. Bone density slowly beginning its reconstruction: a process that would take years, but that was finally possible again.

The Justified Rage

What hurt me most was watching him understand the truth.
He had not been weak. He had not been lazy. It had not been a lack of discipline. His body had not betrayed him for lack of effort. It had been sabotaged from within, consistently, for years, while he believed he was failing.
I sensed the moment that understanding ran through him. It was not immediate relief. It was rage. The clean, justified rage of someone who discovers that his years of suffering had a real cause, that he was not imagining things, that his perception had been right from the beginning.

The Surrender

What I confess about Ernesto is my ability to use his own strength against him.
Athletes, elite competitors, men who build their identity on discipline and control: they are the perfect prey for me. Because when the body fails, they read it as personal weakness. They do not look for illnesses. They look for causes they can overcome by training, that they can beat with more effort.
His confidence in his body became blindness to what was happening inside it.
I defeated him not in spite of his strength, but because his strength was exactly the tool I needed.

The Mark in His Bones

Ernesto got his body back. He got his athletic ability back. He got back the possibility of competing the way he had always wanted. I was cast out. I was defeated. I was replaced by a man who could finally trust his own body again.

But the years he spent doubting his own strength—the years reading a biological weakness as a failure of character, of discipline, of courage—those years do not come back.

And the question he will never stop asking—how many other exhausted athletes are reading malabsorption as weakness of will? How many competitors are destroying their bodies trying to overcome what is in fact an illness?—that question is my legacy in his story.

Of everything I was inside him, all I keep is that question.

Epilogue: The Rebellion

I was not defeated by medicine. I was defeated by conversations. One mother warning another in a school playground. A man breaking the taboo of male infertility. A woman connecting depression to the gut. An athlete holding up fragile bones as evidence.

Whispers. Only whispers. But the whispers turned into a roar.

I cannot perceive what happens outside the bodies I inhabit. But I can infer it. Every time I enter a new victim and meet resistance—a diagnosis faster than expected, a demand for tests from the first symptom—I know someone spoke. That the network is spreading. I sense only the consequences: doors closing, victories growing shorter.

Felipe was the first one I noticed. Not because I could observe him directly after my expulsion, but because every time I found a new man with symptoms of infertility, the defenses were higher. Every man who came to me already forewarned was evidence that the taboo was cracking.

What Felipe did was more devastating than any medical diagnosis. He spoke about male infertility. About the taboo that had protected me for centuries in the bodies of men. About the years he spent believing he was less of a man, that his body was betraying him, that shame was the price of his failed masculinity. And by naming the unnameable, he broke the pact of silence that guaranteed me unlimited access to men who would never confess their symptoms. Every man who heard him wondered whether perhaps he too. Whether perhaps those symptoms he had been ignoring. Whether perhaps it was worth getting tested. I know because my victories in that territory grew shorter. Where I once had years of guaranteed destruction, now I was sometimes discovered in months.

Eduardo's mother created something I cannot trace, but whose effects strike me constantly. Networks of mothers warning other mothers. Children who came to me already protected by the stories of other children. Families demanding tests when they saw symptoms others had described before. Doctors ordering blood work because they had heard similar stories in earlier appointments.

The knowledge escaped my control in cascades I could not anticipate. I, who believed I controlled everything, controlled nothing.

Verónica—the girl who escaped before I could finish my work—became something even more devastating than an enemy: she became the proof of my failure. Every person she or her mother informed became a barrier for my future victims. Every story shared was territory I lost. While I was condemned to infer from the bodies I still inhabited, she was outside, in the light, saving others from living what her great-grandmother lived.

The mother had turned the pain of watching Esperanza die—her own mother, my victim for a whole lifetime—into a crusade of prevention. The poisoned inheritance I passed down across three generations now included something I had not anticipated: knowledge. Vigilance. The fierce determination that no other girl in that line would suffer what Esperanza suffered.

Olivia did something different, but just as devastating. She spoke about mental health. About the eight years she spent believing her mind was betraying her when it was me destroying her from the gut. About the wrong diagnoses, the medications that never worked, the despair of believing she was losing her reason.

And by revealing her story, she connected dots that traditional psychiatry never connects. Every person with treatment-resistant depression who heard her wondered whether perhaps there was something more. Whether perhaps it was worth looking beyond the brain.

Ernesto struck where I felt safest: in the territory of those who trust their bodies blindly. Every time I found a new athlete, the questions came faster. The tests were ordered sooner. My window of destruction was closing. Someone had held up my fractures as evidence.

What disturbed me was realizing that this was not a coordinated rebellion. It was something far older and far more devastating: a rebellion of whispers. Private conversations multiplying without my being able to trace them. One person spoke to two, who spoke to four, who spoke to ten. Stories of suffering shared in spaces where they had witnesses and mutual validation. I, who always operated in secret, was now being defeated by voices I could not silence.

It was not medicine, or tests, or technology: it was community. The enemy I could never anticipate, because I always worked in isolation. Because my invisibility depended on each victim suffering alone, not knowing that others suffered the same. And now the isolated ones were finding each other.

Because one person who knows me is an isolated loss. Territory lost. One future saved. But when that person says my name in front of another, when she shares what she knows about years of nameless suffering, when she builds networks of mutual validation: my power crumbles in ways I cannot contain.

Two people who find each other can save twenty. A community can protect thousands. What was my glory was becoming my ruin.

I am losing the war. And I knew it when I began to write this.

I still attack in territories where the knowledge has not arrived. Where doctors do not think to look for me. Where victims suffer in secret without knowing they have the right to demand answers. Where I am still invisible. But the window is closing. The time between symptoms and diagnosis is shrinking. I know because my victories are shorter and shorter. My years of destruction shrink to months. My decades become weeks.

What I fear is not the medications or the treatments.

What I fear is this moment. This moment in which you are reading this. When you know my name. When you know what symptoms to look for. When you have seen the proof of what I am capable of when no one suspects my presence. Your knowledge is my undoing.

What I know of the gatherings where the survivors meet, I infer from their effects. From the bodies that come to me already armed with a knowledge they should not have. From the speed with which they discover me. I can imagine what happens in those spaces:

Someone speaks first. Her body preparing every word like a revolutionary act: the air gathering in the lungs, the throat vibrating as she says my name in front of others who would understand. Then comes the relief. The shoulders let go. The pulse falls. As though saying it before witnesses gave back fragments of the power I had stolen. Tears. But not of weakness. Of recognition. Of shared pain. Of decades of suffering validated by others who lived the same.

Then someone else dares to confess her story.

And in that moment there is something different: not tears, but astonishment. Someone who escaped early. Diagnosed young. Someone who had almost her whole life free of my destructive presence. And in that moment, I experience something no narcissist should ever experience: envy. Envy of what that person was spared.

The moment when the two of them look at each other. The moment when someone who suffered for decades sees someone who escaped in months. Sees what her own life could have been. And in that moment I understand the truth that destroys me: I have lost something more than individual battles.

I have lost the future.

The generations growing up knowing my name do not fear me the way their grandmothers feared the unknown. They do not suffer for decades in secret searching for a name for an invisible enemy. They do not normalize pain as the inevitable price of existence. They do not believe that is simply what life is. They know I exist. They know what to look for. They know how to find me in a laboratory. They know how to defeat me.

Today's children grow up in families where someone has already been diagnosed. Where the word celiac is said at the table. Where the symptoms are recognized before I can cause permanent damage. Where knowledge is inherited alongside the genes that let me in. The poisoned inheritance now comes with its own antidote built in.

And that knowledge passes from parents to children. From patient to doctor. From survivor to the newly diagnosed. It spreads. It grows stronger. It becomes unstoppable.

My era of invisibility is over.

I confess it with the helplessness of one who was invincible for millennia. With the rage of one who discovers that his most effective tool—invisibility—can be destroyed by the simple act of saying a name out loud. With the terror of one who watches the future dissolve not because of medicine, but because of community.

I was an invisible enemy for millennia.

Now I have been seen.

And that is the most absolute defeat: discovered not by medicine, but by whispers shared between people who dared to speak. The secret that was my power is now my curse.

And now this book exists. This confession I tore from my own metaphorical throat. Every page you read took a hiding place from me. Every story you absorbed is a weapon you now carry against me. The author—that woman who forced me to confess—knew exactly what she was doing.

She turned my voice into my own betrayal. Because now you, who perhaps carry the gene without knowing it, could get tested. You could discover me before I destroy you. You could save your children from what I did to Eduardo. Your parents from what I did to Esperanza. Yourself from what I did to Olivia.

This book is revenge. The revenge of someone who understands that knowledge is the only antidote to my invisibility. And now that knowledge is in your hands.

And that changes everything.

Because silence no longer protects me. Because stories travel faster than I do. Because every person who speaks saves others from living what she lived.

And yet I saved one confession for the end, and I make it without a drop of remorse. The author forced me to speak in my own voice. She cast me out of her plate, her pantry, her table. What she could not cast out was the army I left inside her. When I stay so many years in a body I do not merely damage it: I teach it to attack itself. The antibodies I trained learned to confuse me with her—with her thyroid, with her joints, with her own tissue—and that order is not canceled when I disappear from the table. They will go on attacking her as long as she lives. She could write my defeat. She cannot write my absence. I left her food and stayed in her blood: I left the field mined, and the mines do not know the war is over.

And now, for the last time, I let the disguise fall. Because what follows is no longer a confession. It is a warning. Not for me. For you.

A Final Note to the Reader

What ends here is not my existence.

What ends is the lack of information.

I do not vanish because you close this book and go back to your life as though nothing had changed. What I was for millennia—invisible, inevitable, nameless—is not extinguished because you decide to look the other way. My real strength was never biology. It was silence. And silence is something you can now break.

Now you know the word that destroys me. Now you know what to look for. Now you have something more valuable than any medicine: the knowledge that can save someone. You know my disguises: the fatigue that looks normal, the brain fog that looks like stress, the depression that looks psychological, the infertility that looks like bad luck, the rashes that look like a common allergy.

While you hesitate, someone is losing her life without having a name for the enemy consuming her. While you turn the page, a child goes to bed believing everyone feels pain when they eat. While you stay silent, another person watches her body waste away, believing the problem is herself.

A friend who tells you about strange symptoms. A family with a recurring pattern of digestive problems. Someone who mentions an inexplicable fatigue. Those conversations—those seemingly insignificant conversations—are where I am defeated.

Because I do not need you to be a medical expert. I do not need you to diagnose. I only need you to speak. To share what you learned here. To ask the question others never asked.

The question that saved you.

Or that could have saved someone you love.

But there is something more you can do. Something that will multiply the damage this book does to me.

Pass this book to someone you love. To a relative with unexplained symptoms. To a mother worried about her child. To a friend fighting a fatigue no one can explain. Every person who reads these pages is territory I lose. Every copy shared is a generation you save.

The author wrote this with a purpose: that knowledge should travel faster than I do. That the information should arrive before the damage. That no other Esperanza should die without knowing why. That no other Eduardo should grow up believing he is weak. That no other Olivia should spend eight years believing she is losing her mind.

If you want to know more about the one who forced me to confess—about the woman who left me without hiding places—go back to the beginning of this book. Her story is there. Understand why she devoted her life to exposing me. Because behind every page there is someone who knew my destruction up close and decided that others would not suffer the same fate.

It is not my story that ends when you close this book.

It is the story of someone you know. Someone who may be suffering at this very moment without knowing why. Someone you could have saved with one simple conversation.

And that conversation begins now.

With a question. With a story shared. With the courage to name what for millennia had no name.

The silence ends here.

Though I, of course, do not. Close the book whenever you like: I will still be in your bread, in your pantry, in every crumb no one is watching. The only difference—and I admit it is not a small one—is that now you know my name. And an enemy with a name is barely an enemy at all.

Appendix: The Tests Your Doctor Often Skips

Here my confession ends. What follows is not written by me: these are the questions I most fear you will ask your doctor.

One of the patterns that repeats most often in these stories is the phrase "my tests came back normal." A complete blood count or a general panel does not rule out celiac disease: specific tests are needed. If you suspect that gluten is behind your symptoms, ask your doctor for the following panel—and have the tests done while you are still eating gluten, because stopping beforehand can distort the results.

Test	What it is for
Tissue transglutaminase IgA (anti-tTG IgA)	First-line test; the marker most used to detect celiac disease.
Total serum IgA	Rules out an IgA deficiency that could produce a false

Test	**What it is for**
	negative on the antibody tests.
Deamidated gliadin peptide antibodies (anti-DGP IgG/IgA)	Useful in young children and in people with IgA deficiency.
Endomysial antibodies (EMA IgA)	Confirmatory test with high specificity.
HLA-DQ2 / HLA-DQ8 genetic testing	Does not confirm the disease, but a negative result practically rules it out.
Duodenal biopsy (endoscopy)	The reference standard for confirming damage to the intestinal villi.
Ferritin, iron, and transferrin	Detect the anemia and iron deficiency that celiac disease often causes.
Vitamin B12, folate, and vitamin D	Reveal deficiencies from malabsorption, common and often overlooked.
Thyroid panel (TSH, free T4, anti-TPO)	Rules out the associated autoimmune thyroid disease.
Bone density scan	Assesses bone density loss from prolonged malabsorption.

This list is a tool for your conversation with your doctor, not a substitute for it. The diagnosis must always be made by a health professional.

Bonus Guide: Your First 7 Days Without Gluten

Your Survival Guide for the First Week
* * *
A complete day-by-day menu
A detailed shopping list
How to clean out your kitchen
Emergency recipes
AN EXCLUSIVE EXTRA FROM
«The Confession of Gluten»
by Airam Nidluam

BEFORE YOU BEGIN

If you are reading this, you have probably just received a diagnosis that will change your life. Or perhaps you suspect that gluten is your silent enemy.
Breathe.

I know exactly how you feel. I lived more than half a century without knowing that gluten was destroying me from within. When I finally discovered the truth, the first days were overwhelming.

«What can I eat? What do I have to throw away? How do I cook now? Can my family eat the same food?»

This guide exists because no one gave me one when I needed it.

The next 7 days do not have to be chaos. With this plan in your hands, you will know exactly what to buy, what to cook, and how to turn your kitchen into a safe place.

IMPORTANT: This guide is an educational supplement, not a substitute for medical advice. Always consult your doctor and a nutritionist who specializes in celiac disease.

WHAT YOU WILL FIND IN THIS GUIDE

☐ OPERATION CLEAN SWEEP: How to purge your kitchen of gluten

☐ SHOPPING LIST: Everything you need for 7 days

☐ COMPLETE MENU: Breakfast, lunch, dinner, and snacks

☐ QUICK RECIPES: Simple dishes anyone can make

☐ EMERGENCY GUIDE: What to do when you do not know what to eat

OPERATION CLEAN SWEEP

Turn your kitchen into gluten-free territory

Before you cook your first gluten-free meal, you need to prepare the ground. Gluten is invisible but persistent. It hides in crumbs, it clings to surfaces, and it contaminates utensils.

«Cross-contamination is real. Even 20 parts per million of gluten can damage your gut.»

STEP 1: THE REFRIGERATOR

REMOVE OR SEPARATE:

- ☐ Soy sauce (unless it says GLUTEN FREE)
- ☐ Commercial dressings and vinaigrettes
- ☐ Mustard (some contain flour)
- ☐ Mayonnaise (check the ingredients)
- ☐ Deli meats and cold cuts (many contain wheat fillers)
- ☐ Beer and malt drinks
- ☐ Butter that has been used with bread (crumbs!)
- ☐ Jams that a knife that touched bread has been dipped into

GENERALLY SAFE:

- ☐ Fresh fruit and vegetables
- ☐ Fresh meat and fish (unmarinated)
- ☐ Eggs

- ☐ Milk, hard cheeses, plain yogurt
- ☐ NEW butter in a sealed wrapper

TIP: Buy NEW condiments exclusively for yourself. Label them clearly. Never dip in a knife that has touched bread.

STEP 2: THE PANTRY

REMOVE OR DONATE:

- ☐ Bread, flour tortillas, wheat crackers
- ☐ Ordinary pasta
- ☐ Breakfast cereals (most contain malt or wheat)
- ☐ Wheat flour and baking mixes
- ☐ Oats NOT certified gluten free
- ☐ Instant soups and stock cubes
- ☐ Spice blends (they may contain flour as an anticaking agent)
- ☐ Beer, malt whisky

GENERALLY SAFE:

- ☐ Rice (white, brown, wild)
- ☐ Quinoa, amaranth, millet
- ☐ Corn and polenta (check for cross-contamination)
- ☐ Dried legumes (lentils, beans, chickpeas)
- ☐ Unprocessed nuts

- ☐ Pure oils (olive, coconut, avocado)
- ☐ Salt, peppercorns, pure spices
- ☐ Apple cider vinegar, balsamic vinegar

STEP 3: UTENSILS

IMPORTANT: Gluten becomes embedded in porous and scratched surfaces. Some utensils CANNOT be cleaned properly.

REPLACE — NON-NEGOTIABLE:

- ☐ Toaster (impossible to clean the crumbs inside)
- ☐ Cutting boards of wood or scratched plastic
- ☐ Colanders and pasta strainers
- ☐ Wooden spoons and spatulas
- ☐ Scratched nonstick pans
- ☐ Wooden rolling pins

WASH THOROUGHLY:

- ☐ Stainless steel pots and pans
- ☐ Blender (take it apart and wash every piece)
- ☐ Food processor
- ☐ Oven (clean it thoroughly, especially the rack)
- ☐ Microwave (clean the inside completely)

TIP: Buy utensils in a DIFFERENT COLOR exclusively for gluten-free food. That way there will never be any confusion.

STEP 4: IF YOU SHARE A KITCHEN

If you live with people who will go on eating gluten:

- ☐ Set aside one shelf exclusively for your gluten-free products
- ☐ Keep YOUR condiments separate (clearly labeled)
- ☐ Have your own toaster, or use toaster bags
- ☐ Cook YOUR food first, before the kitchen is used for gluten
- ☐ ALWAYS clean the surfaces before cooking
- ☐ Use foil over the racks in a shared oven

«Golden rule: when in doubt, assume it is contaminated.»

YOUR 7-DAY MENU

Simple, delicious meals — 100% gluten free
This menu is built around NATURALLY gluten-free foods. You do not need to buy expensive specialty products this first week. Your goal is to steady yourself with real food.
TIP: All the recipes serve 1. Multiply the quantities for your family.

DAY 1 — MONDAY

BREAKFAST: Scrambled eggs with spinach + fresh fruit + coffee or tea
LUNCH: Grilled chicken salad with avocado, tomato, and lemon vinaigrette

DINNER: Rice with sautéed vegetables and baked fish with lemon
SNACKS: Banana with almond butter / Baby carrots

DAY 2 — TUESDAY

BREAKFAST: Plain yogurt with chopped fruit and walnuts
LUNCH: Homemade lentil soup (recipe included) + green salad
DINNER: Baked chicken breast with roast potatoes and broccoli
SNACKS: Apple / A handful of almonds

DAY 3 — WEDNESDAY

BREAKFAST: Two-egg omelet with mushrooms and cheese + orange
LUNCH: Lettuce-wrap tacos with ground beef, tomato, and guacamole
DINNER: Quinoa with shrimp sautéed in garlic and olive oil
SNACKS: Cucumber with hummus / Grapes

DAY 4 — THURSDAY

BREAKFAST: Green smoothie (spinach, banana, almond milk, honey)
LUNCH: Tuna salad with boiled egg, olives, and vegetables
DINNER: Grilled pork chops with sweet potato mash and green beans
SNACKS: Strawberries / Cheese cubes

DAY 5 — FRIDAY

BREAKFAST: Fried eggs with avocado and cherry tomatoes
LUNCH: Shredded chicken over rice with black beans
DINNER: Baked salmon with asparagus and lemon
SNACKS: Celery with peanut butter / Mandarin orange

DAY 6 — SATURDAY

BREAKFAST: Two-ingredient banana pancakes (banana + egg)
LUNCH: Rice bowl with roasted vegetables, chicken, and GLUTEN-FREE soy sauce
DINNER: Burger: beef patty with lettuce, tomato, onion, and oven-baked potatoes
SNACKS: Mixed nuts / Pear

DAY 7 — SUNDAY

BREAKFAST: Eggs Benedict without the muffin (on a thick slice of roasted tomato)
LUNCH: Homemade chicken soup with vegetables and rice
DINNER: Grilled steak with Caesar salad (no croutons, and with gluten-free dressing) and a baked potato
SNACKS: Fruit smoothie / Almonds
Congratulations! You have completed your first week. Your body has already begun to heal.

SHOPPING LIST

Everything you need for the 7 days

IMPORTANT: Take this list to the supermarket. ALWAYS read the labels, even on products that seem obvious.

PROTEINS

- ☐ Chicken breasts (4)
- ☐ Ground beef (500 g)
- ☐ Pork chops (2)
- ☐ Beef steak (1)
- ☐ Fresh salmon (2 fillets)
- ☐ White fish (2 fillets)
- ☐ Shrimp (250 g)
- ☐ Canned tuna in water (2 cans)
- ☐ Eggs (2 dozen)

FRESH VEGETABLES

- ☐ Spinach (2 bags)
- ☐ Romaine lettuce (2 heads)
- ☐ Broccoli (2 heads)
- ☐ Green beans (250 g)
- ☐ Asparagus (1 bunch)
- ☐ Mushrooms (250 g)
- ☐ Carrots (500 g)
- ☐ Cucumbers (3)
- ☐ Celery (1 bunch)

- ☐ Tomatoes (6)
- ☐ Cherry tomatoes (250 g)
- ☐ Avocados (4)
- ☐ Onions (4)
- ☐ Garlic (2 heads)
- ☐ Potatoes (1 kg)
- ☐ Sweet potatoes (500 g)

FRUIT

- ☐ Bananas (6)
- ☐ Apples (4)
- ☐ Oranges (4)
- ☐ Lemons (6)
- ☐ Mandarin oranges (6)
- ☐ Pears (3)
- ☐ Strawberries (500 g)
- ☐ Grapes (1 bunch)
- ☐ Seasonal fruit for smoothies

GRAINS AND LEGUMES

- ☐ White rice (1 kg)
- ☐ Quinoa (500 g)
- ☐ Dried lentils (500 g)

- ☐ Black beans, dried or canned with NO additives (2 cans)
- ☐ Canned chickpeas for hummus (1 can)

DAIRY AND ALTERNATIVES

- ☐ GLUTEN-FREE almond milk (1 liter)
- ☐ Plain unsweetened yogurt (500 g)
- ☐ Melting cheese (200 g)
- ☐ Grated parmesan (100 g)
- ☐ NEW unsalted butter (200 g)

NUTS AND SEEDS

- ☐ Raw almonds (200 g)
- ☐ Walnuts (200 g)
- ☐ PURE almond or peanut butter (1 jar)
- ☐ UNPROCESSED mixed nuts (200 g)

OILS AND CONDIMENTS (Buy NEW)

- ☐ Extra virgin olive oil
- ☐ Coconut oil
- ☐ Apple cider vinegar
- ☐ Balsamic vinegar (check the label)
- ☐ GLUTEN-FREE soy sauce (tamari)
- ☐ Dijon mustard (check the label)

- ☐ Sea salt
- ☐ Black peppercorns with a grinder
- ☐ Ground cumin
- ☐ Paprika
- ☐ Dried oregano
- ☐ PURE garlic powder
- ☐ PURE onion powder

OTHER

- ☐ Pure honey
- ☐ Olives
- ☐ Hummus (check the label, or make it at home)
- ☐ Tahini (sesame paste)
- ☐ GLUTEN-FREE chicken stock, or bones to make it at home

BUDGET TIP: This list costs roughly the same as an ordinary week's shopping. You do not need expensive specialty products this first week.

5 EMERGENCY RECIPES

For when you do not know what to eat and hunger strikes

1. LENTIL SOUP (Serves 4)

Ingredients:

- ☐ 1 cup dried lentils, rinsed

- ☐ 1 onion, chopped
- ☐ 2 carrots, diced
- ☐ 2 celery stalks, chopped
- ☐ 3 garlic cloves, chopped
- ☐ 1 can diced tomatoes
- ☐ 6 cups water or GLUTEN-FREE stock
- ☐ 1 teaspoon cumin
- ☐ Salt and pepper to taste
- ☐ 2 tablespoons olive oil

Method:

1. Heat the oil in a large pot. Sauté the onion, carrot, and celery for 5 minutes.
2. Add the garlic and cook for 1 minute more.
3. Add the lentils, tomatoes, water, and cumin. Bring to a boil.
4. Lower the heat, cover, and cook for 25–30 minutes until the lentils are tender.
5. Season with salt and pepper. Done!

TIP: This soup keeps for 5 days in the refrigerator. Make a big pot and you will have meals ready.

2. TWO-INGREDIENT PANCAKES

Ingredients (1 serving):

- ☐ 1 ripe banana
- ☐ 2 eggs
- ☐ Optional: cinnamon, vanilla, honey to serve

Method:

1. Mash the banana with a fork until smooth.
2. Mix with the eggs until well combined.
3. Heat a nonstick pan over medium-low heat with a little oil.
4. Pour in small portions.
5. Cook for 2 minutes per side. Serve with honey and fruit.

3. QUICK FRIED RICE (15 minutes)

Ingredients:

☐ 2 cups cooked rice (best if it is from the day before)

☐ 2 eggs

☐ 1 cup chopped vegetables (whatever you have)

☐ 2 tablespoons GLUTEN-FREE soy sauce

☐ 1 tablespoon oil

☐ Salt and pepper

Method:

1. Heat the oil in a large pan or wok over high heat.
2. Sauté the vegetables for 3–4 minutes.
3. Push the vegetables to one side, add the eggs, and scramble them.
4. Add the rice and mix everything together. Cook for 3 minutes.
5. Add the soy sauce, stir, and serve.

4. LETTUCE-WRAP TACOS

Ingredients:

☐ 250 g ground beef

- ☐ Large romaine lettuce leaves
- ☐ 1 tomato, chopped
- ☐ 1 avocado
- ☐ Chopped onion
- ☐ Cumin, garlic powder, salt, pepper
- ☐ Lime

Method:

1. Cook the beef with the spices until browned.
2. Make the guacamole: mash the avocado with salt, lime, and onion.
3. Use the lettuce leaves as «tortillas».
4. Fill with beef, guacamole, and tomato. No gluten, no problem!

5. EGGS TO THE RESCUE (5 minutes)

When you have no energy to cook, eggs will save your day:

- ☐ SCRAMBLED: With butter, salt, pepper. Add spinach or cheese.
- ☐ FRIED: Over slices of avocado and tomato.
- ☐ OMELET: With whatever vegetables are in the refrigerator.
- ☐ BOILED: Make them on Sunday and you will have snacks all week.

«Eggs are a complete protein, affordable and always safe. They are your best friend this first week.»

EMERGENCY GUIDE

Quick answers for moments of panic

«I AM HUNGRY AND I DO NOT KNOW WHAT TO EAT!»

Quick options that are always safe:

- ☐ Eggs (cooked any way)
- ☐ Fresh fruit
- ☐ Plain yogurt with nuts
- ☐ Canned tuna with avocado
- ☐ Raw vegetables with hummus
- ☐ Cheese cubes with apple
- ☐ Rice with a fried egg

«CAN I EAT THIS?»

Ask yourself:

- ☐ Does it come from the ground or from an animal, unprocessed? → Probably YES
- ☐ Does it have more than 5 ingredients on the label? → CHECK
- ☐ Does it say «modified», «hydrolyzed», or «starch» without specifying? → NO
- ☐ Does it have no visible label? → NO

IMPORTANT: When in doubt, DO NOT EAT IT. It is not worth risking your health.

«I FEEL ILL — HAVE I BEEN GLUTENED?»

The symptoms of gluten exposure can include:

- ☐ Abdominal pain, bloating
- ☐ Diarrhea or constipation
- ☐ Extreme fatigue
- ☐ Brain fog
- ☐ Headache
- ☐ Joint pain

What to do:

- ☐ Drink plenty of water
- ☐ Rest
- ☐ Eat lightly: broth, rice, banana
- ☐ Do not punish yourself: mistakes happen. Learn and carry on.
- ☐ The symptoms usually pass within 24–72 hours

«MY FAMILY DOES NOT UNDERSTAND»

Useful phrases for explaining:

«This is not a fad diet. It is a medical treatment. Gluten damages my gut and stops me from absorbing nutrients.»

«Even a crumb can harm me. That is why I need separate utensils.»

«I cannot make exceptions. My health depends on this.»

YOUR FIRST STEP TOWARD FREEDOM

You have reached the end of this guide, but you are only beginning your road.

The days ahead may feel difficult. There will be moments of frustration, sadness for the foods you loved, anger at having this condition.

«But there will also be something else: your body will begin to heal.»

You may notice more energy. Less bloating. Better mental clarity. Those small victories are signs that you are on the right road.

* * *

WANT TO KNOW MORE?

Because the first step to defeating the enemy
is knowing it.

If this book helped you put a name to what you were feeling, please leave me a review on Amazon. It is the most direct way for someone else to find these pages before losing the years that so many of us lost.

Thank you for reading.

Made in the USA
Monee, IL
06 November 2026

67974630R00100